Abou.

JEAN PAIN is a psychotherapist in private practice. She holds a diploma in hypnosis and psychotherapy and is a Master Practitioner in NLP.

After graduating from Liverpool University, Jean lived in Venezuela for eight years, where her two sons were born. She taught mathematics for five years, then built up her own business in antiquarian books and prints for twenty-five years.

A keen artist and an avid reader of literature and non-fiction, Jean is currently researching the art of creativity. She sees this as a means of furthering a person's belief in themselves and their own powers.

In addition to her busy private practice, Jean lectures and gives consultations at Champneys Health Resort. Feedback from her talks and her wide experience have encouraged her to write this, her first book - a jargon-free guide to her profession for the lay reader.

Jean has three children and three grandsons and lives in Cambridgeshire.

So you think you need Therapy

by

JEAN PAIN

Cartoons by
Charles L Nyman

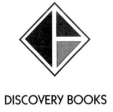

DISCOVERY BOOKS

Dedication

To all my clients from whom I have learned so much.

Acknowledgements

To my family who never fail to give me encouragement and support; to my friends and colleagues Chris Gausden, Robert Weil and Judy Selby-Boothroyd for helping clarify some areas where they are more knowledgeable than I am. To my brother-in-law, Charles Nyman, for the contribution of his cartoons; to my psychoanalyst, Dr Kenneth Lambert, sadly no longer with us, whose powerful influence on my life changed the way I think and enabled me to make the most of my gifts. To Lucy and Alison (not their real names) who gave me permission to use the notes on their case histories. To the publishers Routledge, for allowing me to quote from Bertrand Russell's *Unpopular Essays*, published by Unwin Paperbacks in Great Britain. I also acknowledge The Bertrand Russell Peace Foundation. Above all, to my publisher, Catherine Beattie, for believing in me and all her work to make this book as effective as possible;

First published 1997 by Discovery Books
29 Hacketts Lane Pyrford Woking
Surrey GU22 8PP

A CIP catalogue record for this book is available from
the British Library.
ISBN 0 9518511 8 7

Designed and typeset by David Simpson
Printed and bound in Great Britain
by Biddles Ltd, Guildford and King's Lynn

Contents

Contents

Introduction

This book explains in simple terms what psychotherapy is and how it can improve your life and relationships. I have tried to make it as informative and jargon-free as possible. Psychotherapy is a huge subject and this is not meant to be a comprehensive overview.

Many people are unclear about psychotherapy (some even confuse it with physiotherapy), so I have briefly outlined some of the terms used and explained the basic differences between psychiatry, psychotherapy, psycho-analysis and counselling.

There is much talk these days of 'psychobabble', yet we never hear the terms 'medicobabble' or 'sciencebabble'. Psychotherapy is sometimes derided as 'just talking', imply-ing that speech is too fundamental a part of life to be effective as a therapy. However, when talking involves real communication, as in psychotherapy, it can be very helpful indeed. Every word we speak has an effect on ourselves and on others. Language distinguishes us from the animal kingdom and is the only means we have of crystallising our thoughts. Thoughts lead to attitudes and beliefs. Our attitudes and beliefs affect everything we say and do.

Psychotherapy has the power to help you understand what you really believe about yourself and the world around you, maybe for the first time in your life. This is the first step towards understanding why your life is, or is not satisfactory, and if not, what you can do to change it. When you have read this book, you should have a clearer idea of how the feelings of 'things being right' or ' not being right' have come about. Hopefully, you will realise you have power over your own life. You can take action, whether alone or with professional help to change, if this is what you want and you are prepared to accept the differences it will make in your life.

Whenever an idea is attacked it is usually because it is seen as a threat. Many people fear psychotherapy because they see it as having the power to unsettle old habits. They do not want to admit they are responsible for themselves, blaming fate or other people for what happens to them. They are afraid that their symptoms and behaviour are outside their conscious control and are hiding what they do not wish to acknowledge about themselves.

A healthy mind in a healthy body is brought about by understanding what is going on inside us at an unconscious level and coming to terms with it. The fear of 'looking inside' is often so great that we prefer to believe illness is something that happens to us and is unrelated to the way we live. This belief leads us to look for 'cures' and 'a magic helper' who can wave a wand and make our problems disappear. When we do this, we sell ourselves short by failing to recognise our inner powers to effect our own cures.

Of course, not all illness is avoidable. Sometimes we get ill despite doing everything we can to stay well. There may be some genetic weakness that makes us more vulnerable to disease. It is now widely realised that treating a disease as something separate from the person, as traditional medicine does, is not always helpful. An holistic approach is preferable, as this looks at the person as well as the symptoms and takes into account the mind/body connection.

Attitudes are changing. Psychiatrists, who not so many years ago rejected psychotherapy, can now train as consultant psychotherapists. Many doctors today are reluctant to prescribe medication for depression, without first considering the possibility of psychotherapy.

Symptoms are called psychosomatic when they cannot

be readily diagnosed and are assumed to be caused by psychological factors. If the causes come from within, they can be cured from within. This encourages us to do something about it.

The more you accept the thought that you are the author of your own life, the less will you feel at the mercy of outside events. You will see that it is how you react to what happens that matters, not the event itself. We all see, hear and feel things differently. We can change the ways we look at the world and open up choices for ourselves. We are all unique. There is no such thing as a normal person. Much unhappiness results when people attempt to deny their own inviduality by cramping their lives into straitjackets of conformity.

This book aims to give you a yardstick to clarify the goals of a fulfilled life for yourself. Should you decide to seek therapy it will guide you through the maze of psychotherapeutic resources. You could not be living at a better time. Some of the quickest and most effective ways of solving problems and being aware of our own powers have been developed over the last thirty years.

At the end of the book I have suggested further reading you may find useful. These books are well written, in clear language and are a good read as well as being informative.

Jean Pain

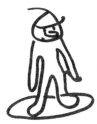

PART ONE
What is psychotherapy?

Psyche is the Greek word for the soul, spirit or mind.
Therapy is the prevention or treatment of disease.
Disease means a lack of ease or illness.

Ease means calmness, relaxation, lack of conflict and freedom from pain. Thus psychotherapy means the prevention or treatment of illness in the mind, spirit or soul.

The best psychotherapy for everyone is the love and care of parents or guardians in the early stages of life.

Love means respecting other people, no matter how young they are, allowing them the space to grow in their own way. It does not mean forcing our own ideas upon them and trying to make them into what they are not.

Many people who come for psychotherapy are suffering from a lack of such nurturing. We cannot change our childhood, but we can learn to understand and accept it. We can, with help, learn to nurture ourselves.

Psychotherapy cannot properly be called a science because it deals with something whose existence cannot be proved scientifically - the mind.

Psychotherapy is an art.

Chapter One

So you think you need therapy?

• *how you can help yourself* • *mind/body connection*

• *what can you get from therapy?* • *common fears*

• *the importance of childhood.*

Why are you considering therapy? Is it because your close relationships always seem to go wrong? Do you feel life is passing by and you do not seem to be getting anywhere? Are you suffering from headaches, backaches or merely feel below par? Is it that you don't enjoy your work and wish to change, yet don't know what you want to do? Perhaps you have been made redundant and cannot find a job however hard you try. Maybe someone you love is sick and you are finding it hard to cope. On the other hand, you may have everything in life to make you happy (or so other people tell you), and yet you still feel miserable.

What can you do to help yourself?

If you have never read any self-help books, go out and buy some now. The reading-list at the end of this book will help. You may have been reading such books for years and even felt some benefits, but the real source of your unease remains. It is one thing to understand a problem and another matter to solve it. Working by yourself has difficulties you may not be aware of. However, we are all capable of coming to terms with certain kinds of personal problems alone. Some of these are described in Chapter Two.

12

It is a good idea to have a medical check-up, especially if you have physical symptoms. Therapists are not usually medically trained, although a competent one will have taken the trouble to acquire some knowledge of how the body works. Nearly all problems of a psychological nature produce some kind of discomfort in the body. It is wise to be sure you are not suffering from an identifiable illness before seeking therapy.

The mind/body connection

Your attitudes and beliefs, the words you use both to yourself and to others profoundly affect your life at every level. When you are at ease with yourself, you don't worry about making mistakes. You please yourself rather than other people. Your optimistic attitude is reflected in your physical health. You will be unlikely to subject yourself to strain because you know when you are tired and take enough rest. Your immune system is strong so you do not easily succumb to infections and viruses. You avoid many of the mysterious aches and pains that come about as a result of inner conflict.

If your doctor cannot find any reason for your physical symptoms, then it is possible your body is reacting adversely to the pressures you are putting on yourself. You are suffering from psychosomatic symptoms. Psychotherapy with the right person could be just what you need.

What can you do to help yourself?

Most people ask their GPs first. There is a difficulty here. Many doctors do not know much about psychotherapy because it is not part of their training. Some are sympathetic to it and others are not. Doctors treat the body as a machine that develops faults, in the same way a car does. Faults are put right by medication or as a last resort, by surgery. A doctor is more likely to refer you to a psychiatrist or a clinical psychologist, because these services are provided on the NHS. The traditional attitude of doctors has been (and to some extent still is) to see illness as an entity, without taking into account the patient's lifestyle and personality.

Psychotherapy is more widely accepted now than it was ten years ago and most psychotherapists advertise. You can look them up in any alternative health publication at the public library or turn to the appropriate section of the *Yellow Pages*. Always check on the qualifications of any therapist you decide to see. A good therapist will expect you to do this.

Action in crisis

So far I have assumed that you have time to consider before deciding to seek help. However, your need for therapy may be urgent. You may be at crisis point. The obvious choice for anyone in a state of despair is the Samaritans who work round the clock. For people with addictions to drugs and alcohol, there are centres in most cities and towns where people with special training are available. Your GP will know about such centres and they are available on the NHS. Alcoholics Anonymous and Gamblers Anonymous are charities staffed by volunteers who understand and have personal experience of these particular problems. They know that their clients need help NOW not in a week's time. They will usually see you without delay.

What can you expect to get from therapy?

Many people who need to talk about their problems are reluctant to share them with friends and relatives. The therapist's professional setting and strict rules of confidentiality give such people the confidence to unburden themselves. This may be the first time in their lives they feel free to speak without fear of disapproval. Many people find they feel much better after the very first session for this reason alone. However this is only the start.

The skilled therapist listens carefully to what you say. His aim is to help you understand how learned attitudes and beliefs affect your feelings and behaviour. You are given the tools to bring about the changes you wish to make.

The therapist is like a detective, hunting for the clues to the real reasons for over-eating, smoking, blushing, claustrophobia - to mention only a few of the many problems encountered. Once the problem has been understood by the therapist, a programme can be worked out to fit individual requirements.

Common fears about therapy

Many people take months to make up their minds before taking the first step of telephoning for a first appointment. Why is this?

There are many reasons. We have no difficulty recognising physical illnesses. Most of us know when our body hurts. Recognising mental distress is not so easy. It creeps up on us gradually. One day you realise you have not enjoyed yourself for some time. You wonder whether this grey feeling is depression. You may not like to think of such a thing. You may be frightened of the term 'mental illness', or even think you are going mad (whatever that means). It might comfort you to know that the definitions of insanity are constantly changing. All human beings do irrational things some of the time. This is normal. Knowledge about how the brain works is still in its infant stages and there are many theories about what 'mental illness' is. No-one knows for sure why human beings behave as they do.

Don't be afraid the therapist will try to make you do something you do not want to do. He or she accepts that you are the expert on yourself. The therapist's job is to listen, respect your wishes, make interpretations and suggestions, which you can accept or refuse if they don't sound right to you.

The importance of childhood memories

In psychology the word 'conflict' means an internal battle between two parts of yourself. For instance, you may have a strong wish to get out of a relationship but at the same time part of you wants to stay in it. The resulting stalemate causes a lot of confusion and distress, as you try to work out what you really want to do. In order to resolve inner conflicts and relieve anxiety and other painful symptoms, it is often necessary to examine and work with early memories. You might be nervous of facing old fears. Are you going to unleash a Pandora's box of old nightmares? Will this be too much for you to cope with? And why is it necessary?

We all carry unfinished business around with us. We may think we have swept it under the carpet, but nothing is ever forgotten in the unconscious mind. Old fears go on affecting us whether we realise it or not. When we have grappled with the 'bad' memories by facing our fears, many symptoms vanish automatically. Phobias can arise because we have secrets we are ashamed of and fear we may reveal them. When you feel you have nothing to hide, life runs more smoothly and you feel at ease and relaxed.

To set forth on this journey of new understandings requires courage and determination. It also requires a degree of sanity above the average. Note that word 'sanity' - it is frequently used to mean 'fitting in with society'. This is not sanity but conformity. True sanity means a healthy mind in a healthy body. It means developing your individuality in the face of pressure to conform. Seeking help when you need to be healthier and more yourself is a very sane thing to do.

Chapter Two

Everyday life problems

• *how to handle difficult situations positively*

• *problems with unknown causes*

• *maturity and balance*

We all have to deal with everyday problems at some stage in our lives. What matters is the way we react to these events. What some people see as a source of misery, others perceive as a challenge. They come out of a difficult situation strengthened, because they are not content to be passive recipients of misfortune. They take control and do something about it.

In order to do this we must first acknowledge our feelings. This does not mean wallowing in self-pity and complaining to friends in a negative way. We won't have any friends left if we do too much of that.

Unfortunately, the repression of emotions in children has been encouraged. 'Big boys don't cry'. We are supposed to be 'good' which usually means not annoying grown-ups. Good is often used as a synonym for 'fitting in'. Some of us grow up so out of touch with our feelings that we no longer know when we are angry, sad or even hungry. Part of every psychotherapist's job is to help a person re-connect with their natural feelings and emotions.

The following tables show ways you can turn your feelings to good account by using them to find a more positive attitude.

Situation	Feeling and its expression	Positive attitude
Bereavement	**Guilt:** Why didn't I go to see him/her more often.	Stop sending flowers to funerals. Send them to the living instead. Make the most of those you love while they are still with you.
	Sadness: I feel sad all the time. I can't stop crying.	Good. Release those tears. Acknowledge your grief. Talk about it to family and friends (don't over do it). You now know what it is to lose a loved one. This experience can expand your understanding of others. The more you grieve the sooner you will feel better.
	Dependence: How am I going to manage without him/her?	Now is your chance. You can begin to find resources you never knew you had. You may need professional help here.

Situation	Feeling and its expression	Positive attitude
Problems with Teenagers	**Guilt:** Where did I go wrong? (Take heart from this. Only caring parents ask this question.)	You did the best you could at the time. Do your best now. Children need to rebel to gain their independence. Stay calm. Don't be browbeaten. Expect them to follow family rules while they are still living with you. Respect yourself and they will respect you.
	Anger: How dare they do this after all I have done for them!	Righteous indignation is useless. You chose to have children and your responsibility is to do your best for them. They owe you nothing. The growing-up years are not easy. Go on caring for them no matter what. This does not mean being a door-mat. By all means let them know how you feel but don't whine or nag. They will protest, argue with you and try to get their own way. Being a parent is hard, the rewards often come later. You can have the last laugh when you see them struggling with their own children.

Situation	Feeling and its expression	Positive attitude
Problems with Teenagers	**Martyrdom:** I suppose I have to put up with all this. I'm only the mother (or father). Don't consider my feelings. I'm worn out with doing everything for you, but don't mind me.	Parents who take this line are trying to make their children feel guilty. Don't do it. They will only resent you. If you have trouble with this, read *Games People Play* by Eric Berne. It will help you get your sense of humour back.
Marriage Problems	**Guilt:** it is all my fault	Looking for blame is a waste of time. Don't bottle up your feelings. Be more open. If you get nowhere, seek professional help.
Retirement (retired person)	**Frustration:** I'm bored. I can't find anything I really want to do. I felt I was somebody when I was working. Now I feel I have no place in the world. Time hangs on my hands.	Tough. It's good to be frustrated. When you can't bear it any longer, you will take action. If you sit around asking yourself what you want to do, you will still be doing that the day you die. Try something - no matter what. You will eventually find something you enjoy. Achieving something, however small, will help you feel less useless.

Situation	Feeling and its expression	Positive attitude
Retirement (retired person's wife/ companion)	**Irritation:** He's under my feet all the time. I want to go out and do things. He wants to stay at home. I would like us to do things together. He watches too much television. He falls asleep in his chair and then wonders why he can't sleep at night.	Don't nag him. He feels bad enough already. Go out and do what you want to do. Go on holiday on your own or with friends. When he sees what fun you are having he may go with you next time. If you have always done too much for him, stop now. Let him fend for himself. He may enjoy the novelty.
Redundancy	**Fear of not finding another job:** Who will employ me at my age? I want to do something different but it's too late. I'd like to start a little business but I'm afraid to take the risk.	Keep all your options open. There are employers who value experience and don't worry about age. It is never too late to start again. Age is an attitude of mind. When you are older you know more and have experienced life. All people have undeveloped gifts they are unaware of. Get some careers counselling. Don't start a business without taking advice or if you are afraid of losing money. Remember, all things worth doing involve taking some risks.

Situation	Feeling and its expression	Positive attitude
Early Achievement of Ambitions	**Apathy:** To reach the pinnacle of success early in life can leave you with a 'so what' feeling. This applies especially to dedicated activities, like winning the Wimbledon Championship. When your life has been dedicated to one goal and you achieve it, you can only decline, unless you change your attitude.	The empty gap in your life needs to be filled by something else. You might find new goals which do not depend on being young and fit. You might try something entirely different which will take your time and attention. Total dedication to one profession is a kind of addiction. The answer is to find a new occupation that gives you a sense of fulfilment.
The Empty Nest	**Sadness and a sense of futility:** A woman who has dedicated her adult years to bringing up a family may well feel useless and depressed when the last child has left home.	See this as an opportunity to make use of your new freedom. Now you might go back to college and train for a new career or polish up old skills. It is never too late to make new friends. The best place to meet compatible people is in an environment where everyone has similar interests. If you have always wanted to do pottery, now's your chance! You have a lot of life left to live. Find out what you like doing best and do lots of it.

Do any of these situations sound familiar? If they do, it may help to take a few moments to write down your present life situation. As you do this, try to become aware of your feelings and listen to the messages you are giving yourself, 'I can't do it', The situation is hopeless', for example. Change the messages to positive ones, such as, 'I can do it' and practise saying the positive statements whenever you remember. Merely repeating the words will have a beneficial effect.

You have more choices than you think. Depression and feelings of helplessness arise when we sense we are stuck. Unstick yourself and you will immediately feel better. We sit in cages of our own making, not realising the door is wide open and that we can walk out whenever we choose. If you were in the middle of a road and a ten-ton lorry was rapidly approaching, you would jump out of the way, unless you were bent on self-destruction.

We can change how we respond to communications and situations we are not happy with. When we do this we break up old patterns of behaviour and see the world differently. You cannot change other people, but you can change the way you perceive them. When the perception changes, other people are no longer the same.

After successful therapy a wife may say 'My husband has changed so much'. What has actually happened is that the wife has changed and the husband no longer relates to her in the old ways.

The times we live in have their own peculiar advantages and disadvantages when compared with the past. Thus we have different expectations, beliefs and problems from our ancestors. Here are a few of them:-

Disadvantages of life today	Advantages of life today
Lack of extended family - loneliness.	Less family interference - more freedom of action
Lack of community life. More frenetic pace of life. Ever-increasing rate of change leading to stress and strain.	Labour-saving equipment - ready-made clothes and food - warm, comfortable houses.
Lack of spiritual beliefs leading to feelings of a lack of purpose in life.	Opportunity to explore many different kinds of belief. More choice - less religious indoctrination.
Too many outside influences making us want what we don'treally need.	Much more freedom of choice in how we spend our money.

Despite the material advantages, there seems to be more anxiety and strain today. Thanks to developments in psychology this century, we are all more conscious of ourselves and more aware of stress.

Some things that bother us would astound our forebears. How do I know who I am? How do I find the ideal partner? How can I find work that I really enjoy? Such questions were irrelevant years ago. It was enough to have food on the table, a roof over your head and a steady job. The key word was 'acceptance'. People expected things to be the way they always had been. Change of all kinds (with the exception of the Industrial Revolution) was so gradual that it was hardly noticed. Few people dared question the status quo. Outside cities and highways, crime was rare. Everyone knew everyone else, so it was hard to get away with anything.

Life has never been easy. Why should it be? We all need challenges to develop skills and creativity. It is well-known that busy people often enjoy their free time more than others. Unrelenting happiness would be dull and tiring. We thrive on variety.

Childhood is a difficult time because our freedom of choice and action is necessarily limited. We have to do what other people say. Children who rebel against their upbringing are more likely to be independent than those who do not. Too much conformity in a child is not desirable in the long term. Deep-seated problems like phobias and paranoia are often caused by an over-willingness to conform to other people's wishes in childhood.

Problems with unknown causes

It may be that you have everything you ever wanted, yet still feel depressed and suffer from mysterious aches and pains that come and go. Pleas from family and friends to 'Cheer up!' and 'Pull yourself together!' do not help. How can you pull yourself together when parts of yourself seem to be all over the place and you can't even find them?

The good news is that every kind of behaviour and symptom has an underlying cause. Finding this can take time and a considerable degree of skill. This is when effective psychotherapy comes into its own. Psychotherapy is developing at a rapid rate and there are methods today that are very beneficial and don't take forever.

Worrying about a disorder can make it appear worse than it is - molehills grow into mountains when we are in a state of fear. Insomniacs often resort to sleeping pills without waiting to let the body sort itself out, which it is perfectly capable of doing. It is surprising how little sleep you need to remain perfectly well. In any event, many poor sleepers vastly overestimate the number of hours they lie awake.

We are all capable of adjusting our beliefs so they are in harmony with our essential natures. When we do this we become stronger, more independent and develop an increasing sense of 'rightness' about the way we live.

The following criteria are my evaluation of what is necessary for anyone to be a mature and fulfilled person:

■ Recognise your worth as a unique being. This includes respecting your own needs and making sure they are met. By respecting your own needs you learn to respect other people's.

■ Discover your innate talents and take steps to develop them.

■ Be aware of your emotions and feelings and stay in touch with them at all times. Learn how to express them appropriately and your relationships will become more open and spontaneous.

■ Have at least one intimate friend, someone you can be yourself with.

■ Have a set of beliefs that give you a sense of purpose. These should be in harmony with your true self, not who you think you ought to be or how other people want you to be.

■ Define your special place in society and make your own personal contribution to the common good.

This is the ideal, something to work towards. The next chapter explains what gets in the way and how the weeds grow.

Chapter Three

How psychological problems develop
- *how defence mechanisms work*
- *coping with life as we grow up*

Imagine you are suddenly propelled into a strange place. A kaleidoscope of colours, sounds and flashing lights revolves around you. One sound pierces through all the others, rising to a crescendo and fading away. What is it? It is your own voice, but you do not know that. You can move but you cannot speak. You do not know what speaking is. You are picked up and gently wrapped in something soft and placed in the arms of a giant who holds you close. You feel warmed and relaxed. The sense of alarm and strangeness slowly fades away. You have begun your journey on this planet.

Your early years
Before you learn words, your mind is in a state of pure unconsciousness. You seem to be part of everything around you. You see something waving in front of your face but do not realise it is your own arm. If someone had given you a book or a map what would you have done? Looked at the colours and shape and put it into your mouth. By the time you were old enough to understand, you would have reached the age of five or six. You cannot protect yourself and are helpless, dependent on the ideas and behaviour of grown-ups.

That is not quite true. You can cry when you are hungry

or in discomfort and hope your message will be understood and responded to. As you grow older, if your needs are not met or you are ill-treated, you have only one resource. You can begin to defend yourself.

How your defence mechanisms come into being

The famous psychologist Freud was the first to use the term 'defence mechanism'. He recognised that much of the inappropriate behaviour he observed in his patients came from a certain way of responding to the world, a way that enabled them to survive difficulties. Everyone's unconscious mind develops unique strategies for this purpose. Here are some of the best known and most common defence mechanisms:-

Denial and repression

Someone in therapy who makes statements such as, 'It didn't happen', 'I had a perfectly happy childhood', or 'My marriage was very happy, we never had a cross word', may be telling the truth or covering up. When the latter is the case, they have succeeded in 'forgetting' what really happened and built an ideal image of how they wished things had been.

Events too painful to face when they happened, have been put aside and the feelings buried. This phenomenon can also be observed in the trials of people accused of committing violent crimes. Defendants appear oblivious to the horror of which they stand accused. They may remain unmoved, whilst evidence is given from recorded tapes by children pleading for mercy. The rest of the court may be in tears. After conviction, they often have no observable reaction at all, or they become very angry, ranting and raving and protesting their innocence. In their own eyes they have done nothing wrong. Serial killers seem to fall into this category. They may have repressed all memory of their attacks on others and genuinely believe they are not at fault. Or they may believe what they did was right, whatever others think.

However, nothing is ever forgotten, and the results of the repressed feelings may make themselves evident in symptoms such as irritability, phobias or depression. Until the buried feelings are brought to the surface and acknowledged, the symptoms will continue.

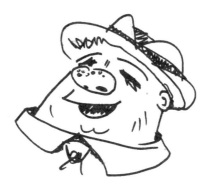

"I do have a drink problem -
I keep spilling it"

People addicted to alcohol may deny they drink to excess. They are not necessarily lying. They may have 'forgotten' whole episodes when they were incapably drunk, and despite evidence to the contrary, insist they drink very little.

Projection

A new-born child does not come into the world suffering from low self-esteem or a lack of confidence. This only happens when the influences imposed upon the child, lead him to believe that parts of his nature are 'bad'. If he is constantly told he is 'naughty', he will eventually believe it and be filled with shame. He will begin to find scapegoats for these 'undesirable' elements. He may blame his brother for something he himself has done. When dealing with children it is better to say, 'That was an unkind thing to do. Look at the trouble you've caused - you must not let it happen again', rather than 'How naughty and wicked you are'. This gives the child an understanding that he can change his own behaviour and that he is not intrinsically 'bad'.

The tendency to blame others is a sign of projection at work. Do you know someone who is always complaining that others are selfish? This is a sure sign of a selfish person. In the same way, people who are devious expect others to be the same and are distrustful of other people's motives.

In marriages, projection is very common and leads to all kinds of problems in communication. A woman who has had a difficult relationship with her father will be likely to project some of her repressed rage against her partner. The same is true of a husband whose mother has been unable to establish an easy, loving relationship with him. He will be quick to notice any tiny thing which reminds him of his mother's behaviour and get upset. It is quite astonishing how people pair up with partners with similar problems. Marital therapy can be very helpful in such cases.

Introjection

It is not possible for us to see another person as he or she really is. We all have an inner picture of our parents and come to certain conclusions about them, because of their actions and how they reveal their feelings. Our inner image of our parents continues to affect us even when we don't see them and after they die. A grown man can be just as frightened of a dominant mother as when he was a small boy. This may prevent him from being assertive with women, making a happy marriage or being able to criticise women employees. He may have a low sense of worth and think he deserved to be punished. On the other hand, a man whose inner picture of his mother is of a helpful and encouraging personality, copes much better with any relationship difficulties he may encounter.

Introjection is a defence mechanism when it conceals aspects of a parent that frighten us. It recreates an ideal image of how the child would have liked the parent to be. Putting people on pedestals comes from an inability to accept the negative aspects of the parent. This hinders our ability to see people realistically. Special people - husbands and wives, children and friends - have to be perfect. People in the grip of the 'perfection spell' often find it impossible to make close relationships because they are frightened of 'making a wrong choice'. Their lives are full of bitter disappointments. The grass is always greener elsewhere. Such people are unable to take risks in relationships or anything else. They are terrified of failure. These inner images of perfectionism and idealisation certainly stop us making mistakes, but they also prevent us from living.

How adult ideas, values and prejudices affect the growing child

When you are a baby, you know nothing of 'right' and 'wrong' or what mistakes are. You do not stay in this delightful state for long. When you begin to draw and colour pictures you have no inhibitions and simply do what comes naturally. Then an adult comes along and comments on what you are doing. The first time someone says you have drawn something 'wrong' your confidence slightly declines. The next time you draw a house, you remember that the walls 'should' be straight, that the windows 'must' have curtains. Too much interference of this kind and you begin to lose your natural joy in doing.

'But,' you may say, 'children cannot be allowed to do exactly as they like. They need to be prevented from harming themselves. To do anything properly, you must learn the rules first. Children have to live in society and must be taught what is right and wrong.' All this is partly true. It is how these social needs are satisfied that makes the difference. Children can be kept safe by placing dangerous objects out of their reach, by supervising them properly so they do not wander off on their own to dangerous places like busy roads. Or you can nag and scold them or even smack them. Children are more likely to behave well and take care of themselves when they are taught with love rather than with fear.

Rules are necessary both in society and in learning skills. The 'right' time to begin learning rules is when ignorance is likely to hold you back. You have to know the Highway Code if you wish to drive safely. Artists cannot paint well without learning the rules for mixing colours, for composition and the use of warm and cool, light and shade. Motivation comes from wanting to do something. Someone who has been made to do something is unlikely to be well-motivated.

There are exceptions of course, but it is nearly always better to learn the rules first and decide later which ones to keep and which to discard. Beethoven once reproved a pupil who had broken some of the rules. 'But you break them' retorted the boy. 'When you have learned the rules as well as I have, then you will know when to break them' replied the composer.

Right or wrong?

There are no absolute rights or wrongs. They vary according-ing to the society you are born into, your family's religious beliefs and many other factors. It is wrong to commit murder, but killing is acceptable during a war. It is amazing how God manages to be on two opposing sides at once. Because something is a common belief, it is not necessarily right. As we become more influenced by outside controls, we learn to 'fit in'. However well-meaning your parents, they have already been influenced by their own upbringing and its prejudices.

What children need

Most people would say love is the best gift a parent can give a child. The word 'love' is used carelessly and means differ-ent things to different people. Some people believe they are showing love by spending money on toys; others think love means pressurising children to do their best. Then there is the phrase 'unconditional love', used to describe the capacity to go on caring for someone whatever they do; not to make judgements nor to expect those we love to fulfil our expectations for them.

Bringing up children requires a high degree of maturity in the parents. Most of us start families while we are still very young and have yet to come to terms with ourselves. We find the arrival of a small being who is totally demanding and self-centred, difficult to manage. We all make mistakes as parents. However, our children will forgive us as long as they feel valued by us for their own sake, not because of what we expect from them.

The best gift we give to our children is to help them become independent from us in stages, at the right time, when they are ready. A good parent allows them to dress themselves when they want and gives them the time and opportunity to develop skills on their own. The child is allowed to express anger, enthusiasm and fear in a safe environment, learning to handle his feelings and deal with them in his own way. Parents need to give reassurance and encouragement without overdoing it. It is all a question of balance, treading the middle path between over-protection and neglect.

The tendency today is to teach children to be too aware of their rights and not aware enough of their responsibilities, the opposite of fifty years ago. What is real morality about? It is not something we force upon our children by lecturing them. It is about setting a good example so our children can learn through imitation.

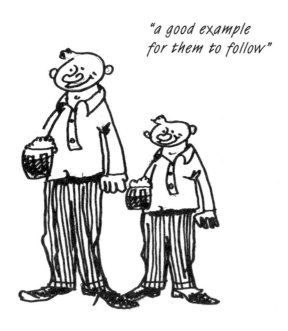

"a good example
for them to follow"

There is often a conflict between fitting into society and satisfying our individual needs, which may lead to an identity crisis. Many people come for therapy for this reason.

The quest for identity

We cannot begin to understand others better without starting with ourselves. Great philosophers and writers have always known this. Shakespeare wrote:-

> *This above all, to thine own self be true*
> *And it must follow as the night the day*
> *Thou cans't not then be false to any man.*

'I need to know who I am,' is a common cry today. It is a healthy sign. It means you are not satisfied with the values you have been taught and those operating in the world around you. You sense you have lost touch with your natural way of seeing, hearing and feeling the world. Your real self feels cramped and cries out in protest. Once you have asked this question there is no turning back. What you seek is peace of mind.

What gets in the way, are all those 'shoulds','oughts' and 'musts'. They are not natural but have been taken on board from the outside. This is because we develop a defence mechanism known as identification. You identify with beliefs from many sources, not only family and culture, but also television, newspapers, books and advertisements. Identification helps you to feel part of society, that you are secure and in step with your peer group.

Unfortunately, the more comfortably we fit into our surroundings, the further we get away from our own individuality. The more we cultivate our unique selves, the more alienated we become. This is one of life's greatest dilemmas. We have to find a middle line to keep the balance between these two extremes and pay a price for our choice. Beethoven is a good example. He chose to be himself and paid the price of sacrificing his personal happiness. Although he longed for love and friendship, his work always came first. He struggled to reconcile this need for other people with his overwhelming desire to develop his talents to his own satisfaction. He plumbed the depths of despair as a result. It is unlikely he could have reached such heights of musical expression if he had not.

A few lucky people have managed to have their cake and eat it. Picasso appeared to satisfy his personal needs and make the most of his talents. He had the ruthlessness of the true artist. People had to fit in with him. It did not matter to him whether society liked his work or not. He went his own way and won acclaim despite opposition. Beethoven also won acclaim despite his originality, but his own moral code towards other people was more demanding than Picasso's, and he suffered as a result.

We are talking about 'great men' here. What about the rest of us? We have exactly the same problem, though on a less exalted plane. If we are going to get anywhere in our personal development and gain satisfaction from this business of living, we have to resist the influences around us wherever they come from. We need to question them and take on board only those that fit in with our real nature.

You are probably asking, 'How do you know what your real nature is?' The answer is to listen to your inner voice. Trust your intuition. If something 'feels good' to you, if it 'rings bells' then it is probably right for you. There is one caveat here. There is another kind of 'feeling right' which can come from an impulse to do something that is not good for us. For instance, listening to a voice that tells you to do what your parents want, when you yearn to be free, may lead you into the position of a self-sacrificing and resentful martyr. There are intuitions which are genuinely yours and others that are other people's. It isn't easy to tell the difference, but it is essential for your wellbeing. Our intrinsic, unique qualities are most evident when we are children, because we haven't had time to hide them. We cover them up because other people don't like or approve of them. If you want to understand yourself better go back to your childhood and remember what excited and moved you. What games did you love playing? Which places do you remember vividly? What did you like or dislike about the adults who governed your life? Such self-questioning will help you to get a better understanding of yourself.

I cannot finish this chapter without mentioning one more important topic, the most important factor in our development. The nature of our brain and how we learn to think.

The left and right brain

The largest section of our brain is divided in two halves, like the two halves of a walnut and of similar appearance. These halves are joined by a complex system of nerves so that they can communicate with each other. Each half fulfils different functions. If you are right-handed your left brain's main function is to analyse or take apart, your right brain to synthesise or put together. The left brain enables us to follow logical structures such as grammar and mathematics. It deals in words. The right brain enables us to grasp things as a whole and make sense of them. It is the brain of intuition and imagination, the brain that comes up with hunches and ideas out of the blue, the brain that enables us to invent something new. It deals in pictures or symbols. Some people think the left brain is the conscious one and the right brain, the unconscious and this would appear to be so. Most of us have been deeply involved in a creative hobby such as reading, painting or writing, when we have been so absorbed that we do not hear someone speaking to us. That is because we are temporarily out of touch with individual words and living in a different world of images and ideas.

Left-handed people have their brain-halves the other way round, so that their left brain is on their right side. This affects them in all kinds of ways that are just beginning to be understood. Left-handed composers, like Rachmaninoff, produce a different kind of music which can be recognised with practice. Some of their phrases sound as though they are back-to-front.

The importance of the senses

All thinking is based on the senses. If we could not hear, see, touch or feel emotions it is doubtful whether we could think. We interpret the world around us through our senses. Thus thinking is not a logical process as many people believe. Our thinking is affected by the way we perceive the world. Our perception is both limited and distorted by the prejudices we have picked up along the way and by our own special interests. In other words we all have different methods of thinking so there is no such thing as a truly objective viewpoint. There are only opinions and theories and all of them are subjective. It is an arguable point whether it is possible to prove anything at all. Therefore it behoves us to start asking questions when we are small and to continue asking them. Obviously we cannot question everything, nor would it be useful to do so. There is a tried and trusted body of wisdom, derived from universal experience which we ignore at our peril. It is better to concede that fire burns, rather than test it out by putting our hands in the flames. However, accepting without question everything grown-ups say, is not good for us, either. Much of the pain we cause ourselves stems from trying to fulfil other people's wishes instead of our own. When we accept that we have the right to follow our own path, we are well on the way to mental health.

Psychotherapy believes in the power of each individual to discover what he or she needs to lead a more meaningful life. Its practice involves great skill; the ability to find clues and make deductions with sensitivity, empathy, intuition, imagination and above all integrity. Psychotherapy does not deal solely with 'problems', nor is it intended to help you 'fit in'. Its purpose is to develop your inner resources so that you can get the most out of life in the way that you want.

Chapter Four

Making relationships
- *the unconscious factors that affect how we choose friends and partners*
- *the phenomenon of 'falling in love'*
- *the advantage of having enemies*

'Give me a child 'til he is seven years old and he is mine for life' said the Jesuits. This statement is only partly true. We are not puppets and we have brains to think with. However it is not easy to change what has been strongly instilled into us at an early age. We all need to remember this, so that we do not impose our own beliefs on our children any more than we can help. The most beneficial effect we have on these little ones, is to set them a good example. When we are non-judgemental and accept each other, our children will tend to follow suit.

How children assess their parents
Children pay attention to what we do, rather than to what we say. They soon notice if you don't keep your promises and have an uncanny knack of noticing your moods and guessing your thoughts. You can make all kinds of mistakes with your children, when they feel secure in your love for them. They will forgive you when they know you value them for themselves. However, should you attempt to satisfy your own needs through them, don't think they won't notice.

How we learn to behave with each other

The first two people we learn to relate to are mother and father. They are our first models for the art of connecting with other people. Later models can be siblings, friends, teachers and other adults. None of them have the same impact on us as our parents or those who take on the parental role. If, when you were a child, your mother was so inconsistent that you never knew how she would behave in a given situation, you might learn to live with her in one of several different ways:-

■ Tell her only what you think she wants to hear (learn the usefulness of lies).

■ Avoid her as much as possible by doing nothing that might attract her attention (learn to distance yourself from those you love to avoid getting hurt).

■ Notice her moods, so you know when it is safe to react to her and when it is not (learn to be watchful and constantly on the defensive).

Later on, when you are grown up, you will apply this 'learned' behaviour to your relationship with your partner or spouse, without realising it. More marital discord arises from this phenomenon than from anything else. This way of relating to another person is called a 'transference' for obvious reasons.

Instead of relating with an open mind to the other person, we transfer to them how we felt about our parents and see meanings in their behaviour which are simply not there. An expression on a partner's face which reminds us of a parent is enough to send us into a rage, leaving the other person bewildered and unhappy.

In therapy, clients transfer old ways of reacting to the

therapist. This can be useful, as the therapist is trained not to take it personally, using the transference situation to help the client understand why he came to behave in that way and what he can do to change.

As 'learned' behaviour takes place at an unconscious level, we are unaware of what we are doing until someone helps us to see it. Our unconscious mind is incredibly quick to pick up new tricks when we are small. There are no limits to its powers.

The unconscious mind - a powerhouse of resources

Your unconscious mind is a vast treasure-house which contains all the elements that go to make you a unique person. It contains records of everything that has happened to you from your beginning. Under hypnosis it is possible to bring back any memory, provided your unconscious mind allows you to do so. Sometimes a memory may be so painful that the unconscious mind waits until you are ready to face it. There is no concept of time in our unconscious mind, so that something that happened in your infancy is revived in all its original vividness when it comes to the surface. The power of these buried images is immense. This is why, when you dream, images arising from different times in your life are not in order. Your dream is taking symbols from your life and presenting them in code form for some hidden reason of its own. The answers to all your difficulties and the resources to deal with them, lie within you.

Nature or nurture?

This is an old argument. Which is more important, what we inherit or the environment in which we are reared? The answer is that both are important, but that our inherited nature is probably the dominant influence. When we look at children in the same family, brought up in a similar way

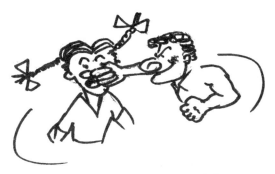

"Some children will fight much harder.."

we notice that one child fights harder to get his own way and another is more acquiescent. Some children are more energetic than others. One child responds to a certain kind of music in which no other member of the family has the least interest. Our genetic inheritance is the raw material on which we build.

How we develop our own particular defence mechanisms depends on our nature. One child reacts to inappropriate handling by throwing tantrums, another withdraws into herself. One grows up with a tendency to criticise others before they have a chance to criticise him, another avoids any kind of confrontation.

How children feel

When we are small we are dependent on the giants who look after us. Their slightest frown is fearful to us. Their anger is terrifying. Their smiles warm us like sunshine. We are at their mercy. We cannot get away from them.

Childhood can be the most magical time of our lives. We feel everything so acutely. Everything is fresh, new and exciting. Our curiosity has no limits. Our imagination works overtime. We have not become jaded by the familiarity of our surroundings.

Sadly, childhood can also be the worst time in our lives. We are at our most powerless. We have to do what others tell us. We bitterly resent the wrongs that are inflicted on us. We invent fantasies about how we can get revenge. Sometimes our fantasies frighten us so much that we dismiss them from our conscious minds and they come out in nightmares. We cannot afford to destroy the very people on whom we are dependent. Small children have not learned to hide their feelings. Anyone who studies them will notice how temperamental they can be. An angry baby can look frighteningly murderous, as can a toddler in a tantrum. In no time at all, this terrible rage may change to cries of joy and delight. Part of growing up is learning to experience all kinds of feelings and to express them in a way that does not hurt other people. Unfortunately, too many children learn that it is safer to hide their feelings and this builds up trouble for later years. Helping people reconnect with their real emotions can take a long time. When the break-through comes, depression lifts and a renewed sense of pleasure in simply being, is experienced. A lot of energy is tied up in repressing feelings. This why depressed people often feel so tired, even though they may be doing very little.

Irrational responses

Bottling up feelings and refusing to acknowledge them, means you are storing up future troubles for yourself. Dormant feelings can erupt at any time. Whenever we over-react to a mildly critical comment or find ourselves flying off the handle at some imagined slight, there is something else going on. The mild criticism, the misunderstood words have acted as triggers to earlier unresolved painful events. The innocent maker of the remarks is often astounded at the reaction and interprets it as a sign of irrationality, illness or incredulity - 'You're not making sense'; 'Are you feeling all right?'; 'What did you think I meant?'. He does not understand. How can he? He does not know your history.

Rational responses

Of course, sometimes there is a good reason for an angry response. When this happens, both parties need to discuss what has happened so that the problem can be sorted out. This is what happens when a customer understandably gets upset over bad service. Bottling up feelings is not helpful. Neither is beating someone up because you don't like what they said.

The importance of acknowledging feelings

It is easier to share your feelings with another if you learned to do this as a child. If you have been told it is 'naughty' to be angry and 'sissy' to cry, it is usually because this is what your parents were taught by their parents. Everyone knows a good cry helps you to feel better. Some couples enjoy quarrelling because they like the joy of making up afterwards. When feelings are not shown, others do not know when you are upset and all kinds of misunderstandings can arise. Children prefer adults to be honest and say how they feel. They become uneasy when a parent glares at them without an explanation or retreats into an injured silence.

How we select our friends and partners

We all need at least one intimate friend. When this is your spouse or partner you are indeed fortunate. People have different ideas about what friendship is. Here are six conditions essential for friendship to exist:

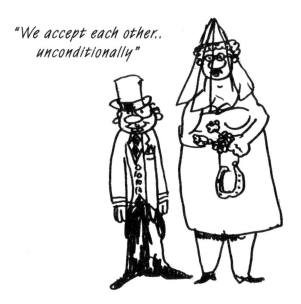

"We accept each other.. unconditionally"

■ Each friend accepts the other unconditionally and refrains from making judgements or trying to change the other.

■ Friends support each other and put themselves out to give help when it is requested and needed.

■ Friends do not offer advice unless it is asked for and even then do so with caution.

■ Friends enjoy each other's company and have similar interests.

■ Friends are not possessive or jealous of their friend's friends.

■ Friends tell each other how they are feeling. They do not have to be 'nice' to each other, yet stay within the boundaries of good manners and consideration for each other..

Acquaintances

An acquaintance is not the same thing as a friend. We may have many acquaintances and very few friends, maybe only one. One is enough. Good friends are hard to find. Acquaintances are people we like but don't wish to get close to.

Many people do not like close relationships because they are frightened of getting too close. These people only have acquaintances, although they call them friends. They are happy to meet, talk and laugh together without getting into any 'deep' subjects. They may enjoy playing games together or meeting at clubs which cater for their shared interests. All of us can enjoy these more lightweight relationships. They demand far less of us and we can take them or leave them.

Keeping up real friendships can be hard work and demands a certain quality of commitment. If you leave it too long before getting in touch with a friend, he may become resentful and think he doesn't matter to you. On the other hand some friendships are so secure that friends may not meet for several years, yet always pick up where they left off with the greatest of ease.

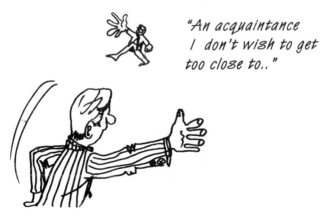

*"An acquaintance
I don't wish to get
too close to.."*

Falling in love

This is a strange phenomenon. Most of us carry around an idealised internal image of our soul-mate. This is essential if we are to fall in love, which can strike like a thunderbolt when least expected. This inner image is like a sparkling, beautiful garment waiting to fit this 'ideal' person. What happens next is outside our conscious control.

You can fall in love anywhere, at any time. You meet someone new and a spark of electricity shoots between you. The beautiful garment you have been putting together with such care has found an owner. In a trice, the person before you is covered from head to foot in an irridescent aura, transforming him into your soul-mate. His skin and eyes take on a special glow. You find yourself irresistibly drifting towards your destiny.

This is the person for you. Your powers of reason are vanquished. No doubt enters your head. Your new love feels the same. He has cast his magic garment over you. This is often a mutual happening, but not always. The beloved may fail to respond. This can be the beginning of a painful time for the lover. Convinced by the 'rightness' of his love, he does all he can to convince his idol that she feels the same. Such persuasion sometimes works. Some people cannot resist being the object of such devotion.

When the attraction happens simultaneously, the lovers go through a rapturous time when they create a little world of two, united so strongly that they feel like one. They cut themselves off from everyone else. They walk on air, hardly needing to sleep or eat, since the food of love is immensely satisfying. They want to know everything about each other. Secretly they wish to be fused together so they never have to part. They are unconsciously in touch with the blissful feeling of symbiosis with their mother when they were babies. They spend fortunes on telephone bills.

To other people, this phenomenon can seem amusing, ridiculous or even irritating. They may smile in sympathy remembering when it happened to them. The lovers do not care. Other people's opinions are of no concern to them. They only have eyes for each other.

Just why do two people choose each other, out of all the possibilities available to them? First, there must be enough similarities between the real person and the idealised inner image. Then there may be a mutually attractive chemistry which sparks off the enchantment, together with a certain charm of body language, tone of voice or expressive eyes.

One thing is certain. This delicious state of affairs cannot last. By its very nature it is ephemeral, like a beautiful rose which must die. Slowly the wondrous garment begins to fade and the real person underneath begins to emerge. The more the lovers see each other, the sooner this happens. Familiarity can breed contempt and destroy illusion. Those who place others on pedestals can easily knock them off, and some people seem to make a speciality of this.

After a while, one of several things happens. If the ideal is too far removed from the reality, the lovers will wonder (when it is all over) what they saw in each other. Or they may be left with a rather special friendship. Sometimes of course, there is a 'happy ending'; the lovers have enough in common to form the foundation of a lasting partnership.

This definition of falling in love does not preclude the possibility that some well-suited people notice their compatibility quickly, even at a first meeting. However, this is felt in a different way from the 'falling in love' state.

There is another kind of first impression reaction. Sometimes we meet someone we instantly dislike.

What's wrong with having enemies?

When we dislike someone on sight, there may be a good reason or none at all. The person may simply remind you of someone else in your life, maybe from your childhood, of whom you had good reason to be wary. In this case, your dislike may be without basis. On the other hand, you may perceive something that annoys or irritates you - the tone of voice, a dictatorial way of speaking or an expression of opinions which clash with your own. This may intimidate you, making you feel nervous. The other person may be so different that you feel unable to establish a rapport with him, dismissing him as someone you don't want to know. You may even pick up vibrations of unconscious hostility from that person. Perhaps he reacted unfavourably to you and you are convinced you don't like him. Of course, you may be quite wrong. I have come across good partnerships and marriages, where the couple involved have admitted to disliking each other on sight, or where one of the pair has felt this way. The initial irritation and friction may prove exhilarating on better acquaintance. There are numerous examples of this in literature and films. A friendship without disagreement soon becomes boring.

We may be right to trust our intuitions. There are some people who seem to be our natural enemies. Anyone who becomes successful, happy or both, will attract enemies because the world is full of envious people. Imitation and envy are the sincerest form of flattery. When you are envied you have arrived!

Envious people identify themselves by refusing to acknowledge that you have achieved the good life by hard work. They tell you how lucky you are. They cannot bear to believe that to attain your aims, you have to take life by the shoulders and shake it up. By blaming their own lack of success on other people or Fate getting in their way, they have an excuse for taking no action to help themselves.

Some people will be your enemies simply because their beliefs are the opposite of yours. These enemies can be useful in helping you see the weak links in your arguments. If you listen to what they say, you may learn from them and even change your mind. You may find that their beliefs are not so different from yours after all. You may simply be using words in a different way with a different understanding of their meaning. When you make the valuable realisation that surface differences are tolerable because you have the same basic values and attitudes, then your enemy may even become your friend.

Chapter Five

Psychotherapy for change

- *do we really want to change?*
- *why psychotherapy?* • *why we stick to our bad habits*
- *the vice of perfectionism* • *the possible effects of change*

Do we really want to change?

There is no point in seeking psychotherapy if we are not willing to make changes within ourselves. If you cannot accept that what troubles you and holds you back may be the result of your own ways of thinking and behaving, then

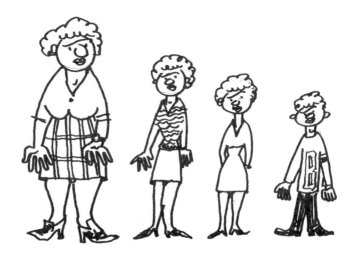

psychotherapy is not for you.

Many changes are inevitable. We cannot avoid growing old, for example. The vast majority of us tend not to change anything until we are forced to. Thus people stay in jobs they don't like and in relationships which harm them. We give ourselves false 'reasons' why we should do this.

'If I keep loving him, he will stop beating me up.'

'If I give her more money, she will do what I want.'

'If I stay in this job long enough I may get a promotion.'

'If I keep buying lottery tickets, I may win enough money to solve my problems.'

There are two great fallacies at work here! First, the assumption that we can change other people, and second, that money will solve our personal problems. As someone once said, money does not make you happy but you can be

"Those who learn from their experiences....and those who don't"

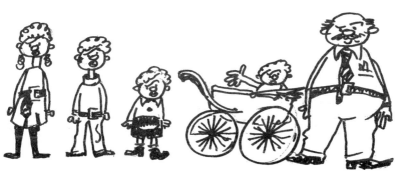

miserable in comfort. Some people think they can get what they want by running away. When you reach your destination and unpack your suitcase, you take out the same unsatisfied self.

When is personal change necessary?
When you feel any or some of the following symptoms, then it is wise to look for professional help:

You get to the point where your life is intolerable; you feel constantly tired, cannot sleep, worry over unimportant things or get irritable too easily; you have problems with your nearest and dearest, feel suicidal, or have aches and pains for which the doctor can find no cause.

Most people do not seek therapy until they are desperate. They may be afraid they are going mad. They think they should be able to sort themselves out. They have probably read self-help books and studied psychology, yet have not found the questions they ought to be asking themselves.

Why psychotherapy?
At its best, psychotherapy can help you change by giving the support you need whilst that change is taking place. Effective, trained psychotherapists know what it is to make internal changes because they have gone through the process themselves and understand it. They can help you summon up the courage to face those things you have swept under the carpet, so that you become reconciled to what has happened in your life and accept it. They know the unconscious mind remembers everything, even events your conscious mind appears to have 'forgotten'. A good mind helps you understand but also rationalises, making it difficult for you to face the truth about what is really bothering you. This is why very bright people are cleverer at fooling themselves than simpler souls. A good therapist is like a

detective, continually searching for clues to hidden causes of all kinds of troubles.

How does it work?

No-one really knows how psychotherapy works. We know that change does not come about by thought alone. We have to change at an emotional level. At some point in therapy we need to release our tears, our fears, our anger, our grief. There is no change without remembering and working through old difficulties. It may not be necessary to remember everything, but it is vital to bring to the surface feelings associated with past traumas. These feelings are so deeply buried that we may find it difficult to believe we feel them at all. However, the evidence lies in our symptoms. Phobias, psychosomatic aches and pains, anxiety and worry may be the price we pay to avoid addressing the real causes of our unhappiness. The important thing to remember, is that we do not produce these symptoms consciously. They are all defence mechanisms dreamed up by our hidden minds. They have helped us survive traumas we could not have faced without them. But why should a symptom suddenly emerge at any time in life? The reason is usually because something has happened to trigger the original painful event. The symptom is a coverup to stop us remembering what we want to forget.

Why we stick to our bad habits?

What we know is safe. We all fear the unknown. Better the devil you know than the one you don't. How can we be sure we are not jumping from the frying-pan into the fire? We cannot be sure. There is no guarantee. All changes involve risk. You are only completely safe when you are in your box, dead.

Anything for a quiet life, is a sure recipe for an unsatisfactory life. Life is not easy, nor has it ever been. If we are over-protected when we are young, we do not have the chance to test ourselves in difficult situations. It is always a good feeling to accept a challenge and win, whether this means facing a bully, working for a degree, leading a normal life when you are disabled, taking part in athletics or enjoying a fulfiled life after surviving a difficult childhood.

The one essential for change is courage. Fear is what holds us back. We need to take risks and enjoy the exhilaration of danger. This does not mean we have to be reckless. We can still use our minds to think things out as thoroughly as possible, but once a decision is taken, we must live with the results.

Perfectionism

To want to be perfect or to do things perfectly is not a virtue - it is a vice. 'Only Allah is perfect,' says the Middle-Eastern carpet weaver to himself as he makes a deliberate error in his design. Being prepared to make mistakes is a great virtue. We all make mistakes when we are learning new things. We learn far more from our mistakes than we do from our successes. Wanting to get things right is the biggest stumbling block to starting something new. The best speakers concentrate on getting their message over as fluently as possible. They do not worry about making mistakes because they know these can be corrected later. Forging ahead requires a confident attitude and the willingness to 'have a go'. Practice makes perfect, provided you know what you are doing. The more you try, the more likely you are to get the results you want.

How change affects us

It is an interesting phenomenon, that when people start reaping the rewards of therapy, they are often unaware this is happening until it is pointed out to them. Things change gradually. An unassertive woman may unexpectedly stand up for herself when she is involved in a car accident. Someone who fears speaking in public, finds he does so unusually well, and that his usual feeling of nerves beforehand has greatly lessened. Someone with a phobia of heights looks out of a high hotel window and realises later that he felt no fear.

Surprisingly, instead of being delighted with the change, some people are uneasy with it at first. 'It didn't feel like me. It felt strange, as though someone else was talking.' People need time to adjust to feeling and behaving differently. The same thing happens when someone moves to a bigger and more beautiful house. At the last minute they may suddenly feel immensely sad and not wish to go, even though this is something they have wanted for a long time. Some people have the same feeling before going on holiday. They may leave packing until the last minute and do it reluctantly. It is only when they have left for the airport and are on their way, that the feeling of reluctance disappears.

Hindsight confirms we made a good decision. When we adjust to the differences in our lives and look back, we remember how awful things used to be and are glad we made changes.

Life is a balancing act. We constantly waver between safety and danger, getting our balance, faltering, then regaining it again. If we never take risks, our lives are stagnant and dull.

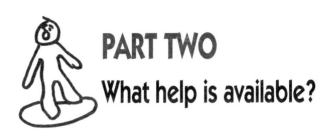

PART TWO

What help is available?

Chapter Six

Madness and sanity

• what is normal? • psychosis and neurosis • criminal or mad?
•are we responsible for our mental health?

---

*'Man is a rational animal - or so at least I've been
told. Throughout a long life, I have looked diligently
for evidence in favour of this statement,
but so far I have not had the good fortune to come
across it, though I have searched in many countries
spread over three continents. On the contrary,
I have seen the world plunging continually further
into madness ....All this is depressing,
but gloom is a depressing emotion. In order to escape
from it, I have been driven to study it, and have
found, as Erasmus found, that folly is perennial
and yet the human race has survived. The follies of
our own times are easier to bear when they are seen
against the background of past follies.'*

Bertrand Russell - Unpopular Essays, p. 82.

Nearly a century ago, the famous psychotherapist Freud
told us that our behaviour is governed by forces of which
we are largely unaware. With hindsight, we often cannot
understand our own actions. Think how many times you
have done or said something and afterwards bitterly regretted it. Why then did we do it? Because we have some inner
and hidden motivation that we do not allow ourselves to

recognise consciously. We may think we want to do something, but underneath, in our unconscious minds, we would rather not. The usual result is that we sabotage our own efforts by delaying or finding some other excuse for not getting on with the task in hand.

Thinking is based on the way we see, hear and feel the world. Without our senses we could not think. Since our senses are influenced by our upbringing and training, they are tainted by prejudices which we often fail to recognise. Thus there is no such thing as purely logical thought. We seek out arguments to support our beliefs. For example, if we need to believe that we love our children, yet reality shows we pressurise them to do what we want, we rationalise our desire to control, by telling ourselves that what we are doing is 'for the child's good'.

Irrational behaviour and deeds only become noticeable when they become extreme. To believe that what happens to you is the result of other people's malice may well make you disliked, but you won't be considered mad. However, if you believe other people are planning to kill you, then you are likely to be labelled paranoid - that is, mentally ill.

What is normal?

One fear that causes people to seek psychotherapy is the terror of 'losing' their minds. Such people may start watching themselves closely for evidence of 'odd' behaviour. They are like hypochondriacs studying a textbook on symptoms, convinced they have every disease under the sun. You do not have to look very far to see strange behaviour all around, every day of your life. One person's 'odd' is another person's 'normal'. There is no such thing as normal. We are all unique. So-called 'mental illness' covers a wide variety of different states from depression or melancholia to extreme forms of behaviour, which used to be called madness.

Psychosis and neurosis

We are all neurotic to some degree. However, most of us suffering from everyday irrationalities are sufficiently in touch with our surroundings to function more or less 'normally'. Those people who have lost touch with reality, so that their bizarre behaviour stands out, are labelled 'mad'. For example, if you are suspicious of others and quarrel with your nearest and dearest, you are neurotic. If your behaviour becomes so extreme that you believe others are out to kill you, you are psychotic. Psychosis used to be called madness. It is psychosis that frightens people. Psychotic people never fear they are going mad, because one of their characteristics is that they think they are right and everyone else is wrong. Thinking you might be going mad and being frightened by the possibility, is a sign of sanity.

Psychosis includes such conditions as schizophrenia, manic depression and extreme paranoia. Because someone has been diagnosed as schizophrenic does not mean they are dangerous to others. However, in a small number of cases they could be. It is as well to remember that we know very little about why and how people become psychotic, and at present it is difficult to treat such people with psychotherapy. This is why the use of medication is so common in psychiatric hospitals. New drug treatments can be effective in diminishing symptoms rapidly, although the down side is that they often have unpleasant side-effects.

It is worth remembering that medical science is constantly revising its criteria for diagnosing mental disorders. New labels are invented to define these disorders more clearly and to differentiate between them. However, this does not mean these illnesses are fully understood. For instance, what does 'road rage' mean?

Criminal or mad?

Much superstition still clings around the idea of madness. Labelling the condition as 'mental illness' has done nothing to lessen the fear - a skunk by any other name would smell as bad. Those diagnosed as schizophrenic or manic depressive are reluctant to admit this when applying for a job, for fear of prejudicing their chances of finding one. The same kind of stigma dogs those who have been in prison. There is a connection in people's minds.

The word 'madness' arouses powerful images of a 'maniac' swinging an axe over his head looking for people to kill. Popular films, like Hitchcock's *Psycho,* have furthered this image. 'Mad' people were once thought to be invaded by evil spirits and this idea dies hard. Where there are criminals and madmen about, watch out! You could be in danger.

In the past, little discrimination was made between criminals and the insane. Both were locked up and ill-treated. Even worse, people went to laugh at the odd antics of the inmates of Bedlam, the infamous mental hospital of the eighteenth century. Parents took their children for a jolly day out to see criminals hanged at Tyburn. We have made some progress since then.

Everyone knows that prisons rarely 'cure' criminals and that mental hospitals rarely 'cure' insanity. People are put away when they are a danger to society or to themselves.

The term 'mental illness' implies a parallel with physical illness, and that it should be treated in the same way. Hence the preference for medication and ECT rather than psychotherapy in the medical profession. Fortunately, this is slowly changing and more doctors are now recommending psychotherapy to their patients.

Kleptomania, sexual abuse, murder and many other kinds of anti-social behaviour are often put down to mental illness. One of the results of this attitude is that criminals are aware they can absolve themselves of responsibility for their actions by claiming that they are mentally ill.

> 'Please officer, the knife just went in.
> 'I don't know how it happened.'
> 'The voices told me to do it.'

It isn't fair to a severely depressed person, to describe his state of mind as the same as someone who has committed a brutal assault on another. No wonder people are afraid to be thought of as mad.

Talking about 'mental illness' encourages people to give up responsibility for themselves and discourages them from realising they can take steps to foster their own recovery, with skilled help. They are led to believe there is some wonder drug to 'make them better'. They may be told there is a chemical imbalance which, when corrected with medication, will effect a cure. This may or may not be the case. There are probably as many people who have not benefited from medication as those that have, and some have been harmed by the side effects.

Why does this chemical imbalance happen in the first instance? We all know of the power of the mind to cause chemical change. We experience it whenever we laugh, cry or get into a state of too much stress. Worry can weaken the immune system and cause stomach ulcers. People with a positive outlook on life are known to recover quicker from operations. If we 'cure' the chemical imbalance but do not look at what caused it in the first place, a recurrence of the same condition is likely to happen. Hypnosis is effective in helping people to give up smoking; however, if the reasons for smoking are not discovered and addressed, the relief will be only temporary.

Electric shock therapy (ECT) is still being used, though

not as much as previously. What a crude and intrusive way to treat a delicate organ like the human brain! The reason for using ECT is because it gives a measure of relief, and when we are in enough pain, we will try anything that might help. Here again, ECT may have side-effects, including loss of short-term memory with long-term memory possibly affected too.

When seeking treatment of any kind, we must always remember that no-one knows everything, that there is no such thing as an 'expert', and that you know more about yourself than anyone else. When you seek help of any kind it always makes sense to be sceptical, to ask questions and not to accept too easily what you are told.

We all like to think there is a magic 'cure' somewhere out there. Remember, no-one can cure us if at some secret inner level, we have a very good reason for not getting well. The care and attenion given to invalids may actually discourage a full return to health, especially if they feel neglected when they are well. True cures come from within the afflicted person. If we believe something will help us, it usually does. However we ought not to take this to extremes, as do some religious sects, who forbid their followers to accept any kind of medical intervention. Obviously if you have acute appendicitis you need an operation. If you have a broken leg it must be properly set by someone who knows what they are doing. Having said that, we need to bear in mind that many types of illness and depression are psychosomatic - the result of faulty thinking and beliefs that cause dissatisfaction in many areas of our lives.They are not imaginary but all too real. The underlying cause is nothing to do with reality, but due to faulty perception. Find the cause, work on it and the symptoms disappear.

The days of miracles are not over. They happen around

us every day. The medical term for them is 'spontaneous remission'. When you work in the field of alternative medicine you soon become aware of the curative power of the imagination, once the will to be well is firmly established. There are many good books on the market which teach the techniques of visualisation and affirmation.

When we treat our own minds and bodies well, by taking care of our real needs (not just what we think we want), and avoid indulging in destructive practices like overeating and worrying, we strengthen our immune system and move towards optimum health.

There is a well-known Chinese saying 'Let your food be your medicine and medicine be your food.' Certainly, there is evidence to show that a simple diet is healthier than one high in chemical additives, sugar and saturated fat. For example, the simple vegetarian and rice diet of many Far Eastern people causes few digestive ailments. Where people are poor and have to do hard physical work on the land to survive, they keep their physical stamina and strong bones for longer than do we in the West.

Since the workings of the body are so complex, it is hardly surprising that sometimes the machinery develops faults. The amazing thing is that everything works perfectly well most of the time, despite how we abuse our bodies and minds. Our genetic inheritance may be our good or bad fortune, but it is what we do with it that matters, and that is our own responsibility.

Medication has its place in the treatment of mental disorders (for want of a better name) and can help ease severe pain temporarily. It is always wise to remember that medication mostly alleviates symptoms *without* getting to the root of the problem.

Depression is a good example. Many people misunderstand what the term means. Doctors use the label 'endogenous depression' to describe feelings which arise without an obvious cause in the patient's life. When someone suffers the death of a loved one, feelings of being in low spirits are normal and to be expected - this is referred to as 'reactive depression'. However, if someone is in poor spirits when everything in their life appears to be going well, the feeling is attributed to a character trait, assumed to be inherited.

Psychotherapists view depression differently, looking instead for some cause in the patient's life - past or present but usually both. Some therapists work in what they call 'the here and now'. However, the present cannot be separated from the past. It is helpful to assume that some unfinished business from the patient's past has been triggered by an apparently insignificant event in the present, releasing buried feelings of discomfort.

Depression is not sadness, although it may contain an element of sadness. Sadness is the expression of a real feeling we all experience during the course of our lives. Depression, as understood by psychotherapists, is a muted sense of being disconnected from life, of being out of touch with our emotions, of not wanting to do anything, of finding it impossible to get any enjoyment out of life. At its worst, depression can cause you to feel as though life has no meaning, that it has nothing to do with you. People who can weep when depressed are not in as deep a state of depression as those who cannot. Tears are healing and release powerful hormones into the bloodstream. This is why we all feel better after a good cry.

Some people feel depressed by all the evil things going on in the world. This is a sign of mental health, not the opposite. However, to allow this to constrict you, is to refuse to acknowledge your own powers. We cannot change the world but we can change ourselves. Any inner changes we make release our powers of creativity and growth and affect the environment around us. When we are doing something, however small, to alleviate our own suffering, we evoke a positive effect on other people. To take action requires great courage. People who seek psychotherapy are acknowledging their own needs and are prepared to do something about it. They are not weaklings. They are peculiarly sane in a neurotic world.

Psychotherapy can be very effective for depression. There are various approaches which will be explored in the next chapter.

Chapter Seven

The talking therapies

• *communication* • *what happens when we talk to another person*

• *the differences between psychoanalysis, psychotherapy and counselling*

• *the importance of language* • *some kinds of talking therapies*

• *two case histories*

When one person speaks to another, he immediately starts to reveal his own personality. Perhaps we all know this at an unconscious level, which is probably why so many of us have difficulty talking to strangers. We are afraid of giving away too much about ourselves to someone we don't know. We fear they might use it against us.

Once we know someone a little better, we open up and speak more freely. We are beginning to know this stranger (it's a lifetime's work getting to know yourself, let alone anyone else). What we mean is that we have some idea of the other person's attitudes and beliefs. We know what *not* to say to avoid treading on their toes.

If we pursue a friendship with this person, all goes well for a while, because we are still careful about what we say, so as not to upset them by conflicting with their beliefs. However, the better we get to know each other, the harder it is to monitor what we say, and sooner or later we feel comfortable enough to speak more freely. Once we do , we give a fuller reign to our unconscious minds and find it harder to control what we are saying. The result is we reveal more of ourselves and so does our friend. Sooner or later we shall be involved in conflict - the inevitable result of two people beginning to get closer. Why? Because we are all unique human beings and if we are being honest with each other, some disagreement is inevitable.

It is how we handle this conflict that determines the outcome of the relationship. If we can tolerate each other's differences and even learn to *enjoy* them, there is a chance we may get closer and become friends. If not, we will part in the self-righteous belief that the other person is at fault, and that somewhere out there is our soul-mate, who will understand us completely so that we can have a 'perfect relationship'.

The truth of the matter is that we all have inner grievances, of which we are largely unaware. They tend to surface in our conversation, especially with those we know well. These are the sum of all the times in our childhood when we felt oppressed, unloved, unsatisfied or undervalued, feelings that have hung around in our unconscious minds because it was not safe to express them when we were small.

It is important to remember that there is no such thing as 'forgetting' the past. Whatever was swept under the carpet and not dealt with can emerge at any time. Do you remember an occasion when you felt furiously angry over something trivial, like someone forgetting your birthday, or chiding you for not returning something you'd borrowed? Nothing terribly important, in fact quite understandable, so why the rage? Something has reminded you of a much greater, buried sense of injury.

When anyone is being particularly difficult over a relatively unimportant issue, it helps to remember it is that person who has the problem. It is not your problem, it is theirs. If you react to their temper by losing your own, matters only get worse. When you realise the anger is not personal to you, you can handle it differently by remaining calm and keeping your own grip on reality. It takes two to quarrel.

All people working therapeutically with others, need to know how to contain and deal with these inevitable expressions of emotion, relating to a person's past. This is known as 'transference'. We transfer onto others all the feelings, good and bad, that remain unresolved from our early life. It happens all the time, and everyone does it to a greater or lesser extent. A certain measure of neurosis makes us human and more able to understand others' difficulties. It is no accident that most good therapists have themselves gone through the mill.

The talking therapies

■ *Psychoanalysis*

It was Freud who initiated what are often called 'The Talking Therapies.' His method was to ask the patient to lie on a couch and then come out with whatever entered his head. The prone position made the patient feel as relaxed as possible and encouraged his thoughts to flow freely. The underlying assumption was that if the patient talked long enough, he would reveal the hidden source of his ills. The same method is used by interrogators, who know that when a person is encouraged to talk, he often gives away his secrets unwittingly.

Freud would listen carefully, saying as little as possible, searching for clues in the language of his patients to help him understand what had happened to them in the past to cause their present discomfort. Psychoanalysis has developed in different ways since then, but the basic principle remains the same. The analyst interrupts as little as possible, restricting himself in his responses, so that the patient comes to his own conclusions in his own time. This is the reason why psychoanalysis can be so lengthy.

As the patient begins to talk, he transfers all his long-standing grievances and unfulfilled longings to his analyst. He may begin to blame his analyst for all the things his father or mother did. He may complain that the analyst is no good and doesn't care about him or he may criticise his mannerisms or even his clothes. On the other hand, he may transfer his own inner idea of the 'perfect parent' and develop strong feelings of devotion towards his analyst. If the patient is a woman and the analyst a man, she may 'fall in love' with him, or vice versa, a male patient may do the same with his woman analyst.

The whole point is that the analyst recognises that none of these feelings are 'real' although they feel real enough to the patient. The patient is expressing his innermost thoughts in emotional form. The patient is not reacting to the analyst because he cannot know him (the Freudian analyst is careful to disclose as little as possible about himself). He acts as a screen on which the patient sees his own nature reflected back to him. The patient is helped to understand the real source of his pain by remembering times in his childhood when he had similar feelings. This enables him to see the connections between old injuries and present behaviour.

Psychoanalysis pre-supposes that if the patient knows too much about the analyst, it interferes with the process and successful completion of the work. Criticism of the therapy from those who have experienced it, is often about the lack of interaction by the analyst. Another criticism is that it takes too long. It could, theoretically, take forever, because no matter how deep the work may be, there is always more to be done.

■ *Analytical psychology*

This is another form of psychoanalysis developed by the psychologist Carl Jung, based on the theory that all people have spiritual needs which must be satisfied. It differs from Freud's method in its underlying ideas and assumptions, but the way it is conducted is very similar with rather more interventions on the part of the therapist.

Psychoanalysts undergo a lengthy training which includes their own personal analysis. Many people think psychoanalysis is a kind of psychotherapy. It is not. There is a general belief that psychoanalysis goes deeper than psychotherapy. This is not necessarily the case.

■ *Differences between psychoanalysis and psychotherapy*

The most notable differences between psychoanalysis and psychotherapy are that psychoanalysis takes far longer, and that in psychotherapy, the therapist has more freedom in establishing rapport with the patient.

Just why does psychoanalysis take so long? The chief reason is that it is unfocused. The analyst waits for the patient to begin to talk. In extreme cases, it is possible for the patient to lie on the couch for months without saying a word, before he can bring himself to break the silence. This is part of the dogma - if the analyst brings up a subject, it may get in the way of the patient saying what he needs to say. It is assumed that the patient needs to attend three to five times each week to keep the continuity of the process going.

Psychotherapy is much more focused. The therapist starts with the patient's symptoms and uses all his knowledge and expertise to discover their underlying causes. The patient is helped to become aware of what he needs to overcome his difficulties and to work at finding ways to satisfy those needs. The patient decides just how deeply he must go to live his life in a more satisfactory way. Psychotherapy is convergent, in that it aims to find clues to close in on the underlying cause. Psychoanalysis is divergent. The patient can go on bringing up material forever, as we never come to an end of understanding our nature and how we function. It is like an author who never gets a book finished because he never feels he has enough material.

The psychotherapist usually interacts more with the patient than the psychoanalyst. He is willing to make disclosures about himself and his own experiences if he feels this benefits the patient. He may start off the session any way he chooses, often by asking the patient what has happened in his life since the last session. He can stop talking when the patient has responded and is ready to take over the talking role. Like the analyst, he keeps his boundaries clear so that the patient begins to appreciate the difference between talking to a professional and talking to a friend. The therapist can use any methods he feels might assist his patient make the necessary connections between past ills and present difficulties. The therapist proceeds with care and chooses his words carefully, as he knows it is impossible for the patient not to be influenced, non-verbally as well as verbally. His role is to facilitate and it is not appropriate for him to impose his own ideas on the patient.

Psychotherapy and counselling

Psychotherapy and counselling are closely linked. The term 'counselling' was coined by Carl Rogers in America. Although he was an academic he did not possess the necessary medical qualifications to allow him to practise in California. He had to call himself something other than a psychotherapist so he chose to be a counsellor. He developed his own methods which are highly valued today. They depend on the establishment of a close rapport between the counsellor and patient which is in turn dependent upon the honesty and 'realness' of the counsellor. The therapist aims at being himself, not assuming some artificial role, and being open and receptive to the patient's needs.

In the U.K. there is counselling training and psychotherapy training, with no clearly defined differences. Similar skills are taught for both methods.

Psychotherapy is an umbrella term covering many different kinds of work. Until quite recently, psychotherapy, as distinct from psychiatry was not recognised by the medical profession. Most training was organised outside the public sector and standards ranged from excellent to mediocre. However, the best kinds of training began to produce therapists who were so effective in their work that the value of psychotherapy gradually became recognised. This influenced the medical profession to start training some of their psychiatrists in psychotherapy. Up to that time, psychiatrists had worked mostly from the medical model, assuming that mental disorders occurred like physical illnesses and were best treated with medication and ECT.

Now, the whole scene is changing and many more colleges and universities provide courses in psychotherapy and counselling. Different methods of psychotherapy are undertaken by the private sector and by the psychology departments of some universities.

▓ *Two different approaches to psychotherapy*
In psychotherapy, we can work from the outside to the inside or the inside to the outside. We can work on the behaviour itself (the symptoms) and try to remove what is causing them (the behavioural approach). Alternatively, we can go straight for the underlying causes, hoping that when these are dealt with, the behaviour will change spontaneously (the psychodynamic approach).

The behavioural approach is easier to use, as it does not require insight and uses techniques like visualisation. It is as though, by changing the clothes you change the person inside them. It works from the outside to the inside.

The psychodynamic approach works directly on the underlying cause of the behaviour. It assumes that if the patient understands and comes to terms with his hidden and often long-standing traumas, then the uncomfortable symptoms will disappear and his attitude to life will change. This approach is dependent on the therapist's imagination, intuition and ability to 'get on the same wavelength' as the patient. This is working from the inside to the outside. It requires far more skill than the behavioural approach because it works at much deeper levels of the human mind.

These two approaches are at opposite ends of the spectrum. Both could be said to be right because we are more than just machines. We can programme and re-programme ourselves. We have free will.

Phobias can be resolved by both approaches. If I have a patient who suffers panic attacks when in an enclosed space and must sit next to an exit door, I can use de-sensitisation techniques. I get her to face the fear by going into the situation - first, by using her imagination and then, by actually doing what she fears. Or I can work directly on helping her discover the associations between her present fears and past traumas. Both methods produce good results but the psychodynamic method is likely to have a more lasting effect. However, this does not have to be an 'either or' situation. It is possible to find a balance between the two extremes by using parts of each method. Habits are hard to break and even when we know why we have developed them, it usually takes some time before change takes place. The behavioural approach can be helpful here.

■ *Cognitive therapy*

Cognitive therapy is very popular. It is a kind of behaviour therapy, because it tackles directly the underlying thoughts, daydreams and attitudes of patients by examining their language. There is a direct interchange between therapist and client. Clients are not encouraged to talk at length about their problems, but are shown how their words reflect attitudes and influence behaviour. They are helped to change their language and the thinking behind it. They learn to become more positive by giving different meanings to experiences and recognising their power to change how they react to situations. They are asked to do homework between sessions and their progress is measured on charts. Cognitive therapy is a 'here and now' method. It may not take into account how the ways of thinking have come about.

■ *Neuro-linguistic programming (NLP)*

NLP has deservedly become popular because it is effective in many fields as a way of improving communication. It is used extensively in business training to build up confidence and show people how they can influence others and enhance their performance. NLP's great popularity is due to the fact that it appeals to both scientific and arts-orientated people and because it is possible to get quick results with certain types of cases. Its approach is logically and clearly defined and exceptionally positive. It takes into account both sides of the brain and all the senses, linking them up in helpful ways

NLP tends to be thought of as a behavioural method. In fact it can work psychodynamically. You can be led back through time to help you to get in touch with earlier traumas. Techniques are then used to enable you to experience your past differently. This lessens the stranglehold of old fears, changing the pernicious effect of those traumas so that your present life is no longer held back. In America, useful work has been done with Vietnam war veterans who have made good recoveries after their buried memories of severe battle traumas have been worked through.

NLP can work with astonishing speed for certain kinds of phobias. It gives quick results for other types of problems too. However, there are always cases where the process needs to be long term and cannot be hurried, whatever the techniques used. It depends not only on the effectiveness of the therapist, but on the nature of the problem and the character of the client.

NLP has a great appeal to both scientifically and arts orientated people, as its approach is logical and clearly defined and it takes into account the use of all the senses as well as the right and left brain. Ericksonian Hypnosis is an important part of NLP. Its success owes much to its effectiveness in teaching communication skills at every level and in all areas of life.

■ *Gestalt therapy*

Gestalt therapy is based on the theory that all our needs are satisfied when we successfully complete the full cycle of our activities. For example, when we are bereaved, we need to work right through the experience and leave it behind. All our ills are assumed to be caused by unfinished business (uncompleted cycles from the past). Thus the aim of the therapy is to discover exactly at what point in the cycle we become stuck.

Someone who cannot give up mourning has not learned to let go, someone who has trouble with procrastination finds getting started diffcult, someone who overeats has not learned when he has had enough. Whatever the situation, the cycle always remains uncompleted at the same point.

Some people never start anything easily and have a problem with time in all areas of their lives. Others find they have difficulty in any situation that involves letting go of the past, so they hoard unwanted objects and cling to friends they would be better off without.

Gestalt aims at completing the cycles of unfinished business from the past. Role-playing is encouraged. There is a strong element of drama in this method. It works well in groups where the participants are encouraged to interact. Each person is helped and supported to gain the courage to explore a painful past experience. It is a good method for extroverts, who naturally tend to gravitate towards other people, but also helps shy people by encouraging them to come out of their shells.

■ *Hypnotherapy*

Hypnosis often gets a bad press. People think of it as a way of gaining power over others and getting them to do something they don't want to do. Another common fear is that they will give away secrets they wish to keep to themselves, whilst 'under the influence'.

These are the facts. Hypnosis is just one of many different trance states. We all experience trance states every day. A child bored by a teacher will go into a trance state and not hear a word; as will anyone who 'loses himself' in a book, a television programme, a conversation or anything else that absorbs the attention. We are all suggestible to ideas coming in from outside. The more imaginative and sensitive we are, the more easily we are affected. Meditation and prayer are other examples of trance states.

When we are 'entranced' our conscious minds have less control and the imagination (lodged in our unconscious mind), takes over. This is why we are easily influenced.

Hypnotherapy works well for addictions like smoking,

nail-biting and over-eating. However, in the long-term it is only effective when the underlying reasons for the addictions are addressed. People become addicted because there is some unfulfilled need in their lives. Mere suggestions alone are rarely enough to effect a long-term release from the addiction. We must really want to be free of the habit. A good hypnotherapist will take great pains to listen to the client and find out what it is he really needs and only *then*, use direct suggestions.

The so called 'false memory syndrome' has been given much publicity. Some people are believed to have invented memories whilst undergoing treatment with hypnosis, then convinced themselves that these 'memories' are real. The evidence for this has not been clearly established and is open to question.

A major factor in the success of any therapy is helping a disturbed person remember the traumas causing their discomfort. Symptoms can literally disappear overnight once their source has been uncovered and dealt with.

The hypnotherapist must always be ethical and never suggest ideas to the client. Nor should he ask leading questions, which might make the client believe they have suffered a trauma such as sexual abuse - even if he has picked up enough clues to think it is a possibility. Should you be working with a hypnotherapist who seems to be coercive, making you uncomfortable, tell him how you feel, and if he persists and does not respect your feelings, *leave at once.* Hypnosis is such an effective tool, that it would be unfortunate if someone who could benefit from it, was put off by bad publicity. Remember, any kind of therapy or medicine can be harmful in the hands of an ineffective or unscrupulous practitioner.

We are all capable of being sent into a trance by listening

to the droning voice of someone making a boring speech.
However, when you know someone is attempting to hypno-
tise you, this will only be successful if you co-operate with
the hypnotherapist. The essence of co-operation is trust, so
it is is important to feel comfortable with your hypnotherapist. Hypnosis is a useful tool for the following reasons:

- ✔ Helps you relax your whole body, thus building up
  the strength of your immune system.
- ✔ Speeds up the building of self-confidence,
  making you more aware of your natural talents
  and resources.
- ✔ Helps you get in touch with buried feelings that need
  working through.
- ✔ Frees you from the negative effects of old traumas.
- ✔ Enhances your natural creativity, improving
  your performance in areas of work and play
  where you feel you could do better.

Most of all, hypnosis can be very effective when used at
the end of a consultation to reinforce the work done in the
session and to send the client away feeling good.

■ Client-centred therapy

Developed by Carl Rogers, this method is the basis of most
counselling courses.

It stresses the importance of the therapist/client
relationship as the most important factor in successful
work. Client-centred therapy is rapidly becoming acknowledged by therapists of all persuasions. The therapist must
respect the client's wishes and realise that he knows best
about his own needs. He may want help to discover just
what those needs (as distinct from wants) are. Listening is
considered vitally important and is something not many of
us are very good at. When a client knows you are fully

concentrated on what he is saying, he feels valued and empathy is established.

■ *Transactional analysis*

Transactional analysis (TA) is more popular in America than in the United Kingdom. The method was developed by Dr Eric Berne who wrote the best-selling book *Games People Play.* The work revolves around the following theory. We all play three roles, that of a child, an adult and a parent. A properly mature relationship is one based on adult speaking to adult. However, when, for example, we are in fear of authority, it is easy for us to go into child mode, instead of maintaining our adult status. This makes us vulnerable to domination so that we cannot stand up for ourselves. Through TA we learn to change the way we react in certain situations, so we get a different response from other people and avoid being manipulated by them. TA tells us that we all have a life script formed when we are small children, by influences inside and around us. Thus we devise our own fate for the future. If this fate is an unhelpful one, TA can help us to change it for something more useful.

■ *Eclectic therapy*

Therapy using a mixture of different approaches. Instead of sticking to one method, some therapists prefer to use a combination of different therapies to help the client. This means the client receives 'custom-made' therapy, designed just for his needs. Since everyone is different, this makes good sense.

Sometimes people ask me how I cure people of smoking. I explain that I don't do 'cures', but show my clients how to 'do-it-yourself'. Then with my facilitation and support and their determination and work, they can achieve what they want. I have no set approach to helping someone to stop smoking because every smoker is different and I work with the person rather than the symptom. The enjoyment of being a therapist lies in the challenge of every new client who comes through the door. It is also exciting to keep up-to-date with new trends and learn more ways of helping the client. As in any subject, the more knowledge you have, the better.

This list of therapies is not meant to be comprehensive. Those explained in this chapter are some of the best-known, tried and tested kinds. Something does not become popular if it is worthless. Hopefully you are now clearer about the different types of therapy available and have a better idea of what might suit you. The language we use to ourselves and to others has an enormous influence on our lives. The people we have most effect on are ourselves. The people we have the most power over are ourselves. We cannot change others, but we *can* change ourselves. Then, surprise, surprise, the world changes with us!

Two case histories using eclectic therapy (a combination of different therapies)

Jonathan and the bully

Jonathan and David are two brothers I know well. They are bright, lovable children.who are lucky to be surrounded by adults who love and respect them. This does not prevent them coming up against life's difficulties.

When Jonathan was seven, he became somewhat withdrawn and seemed to lack his usual energy. He would come home from school with his clothes unusually muddy, yet could not give his mother, Alison, a satisfactory reason for this. She asked if I could help.

I invited the boys and their mother round to my house.

Both boys are competitive and enjoy board games, so I thought a game of lotto would loosen things up and get rid of their inhibitions. As they played and began winning and losing, their emotions surfaced. Suddenly Jonathan burst into loud tears. "Whatever's the matter?" I said. "David made a nasty face at me," he sobbed. "Show me that face, David" I requested. When he did so, I burst into loud crying with exaggerated bodily movements of terror. "What a terrible face!" I said. "No wonder you were frightened. Do it again David." David complied, and I responded with an even greater pantomime, falling to the floor and kicking my feet. This time Jonathan did not respond, but looked at me uncertainly for a few moments before starting to laugh. Soon we were all pulling faces and giving exaggerated responses, then howling with laughter. "Come with me, Jonathan" I said, leaving Alison and David to carry on without us.

"Tell me, Jonathan, when did someone look at you like that before?" "At school" he said, "A boy called Johnnie." "Jonathan, how did your coat get muddy?" More tears, followed by "Johnnie kept pushing me over at playtime." I asked him why he hadn't told his teacher. He paused before replying, "I didn't want to tell on him." I asked him if he was afraid, but he shook his head. "Is he a big boy, bigger than you?" I asked. Another shake of the head. "What could you have done to stop him from pushing you over?" "I don't know." "Well, you are a big, strong boy, you could have pushed him back." Floods of tears, "No, I couldn't, I might have hurt him." "Well, he was trying to hurt you, wasn't he? If he knows what it feels like, he won't be so keen to try it next time."

I suggested we played a game where I pretended to be Johnnie, so Jonathan could learn how to respond differently when he was attacked. As expected, at first he found

84

this difficult, but with encouragement and using his good sense of humour, he learned to push back just enough to show resistance without aggression.

He seemed happier and soon became his old self again, no longer coming home covered in mud.

I used a combination of cognitive therapy, NLP and role-playing with Jonathan. Children are in many ways easier to work with than adults because they are less inhibited and more in touch with their imagination and feelings. It is a mistake to ply them with questions first. An oblique approach works best.

"I'm so confused..."

I received the phone call at 10am. "I'm so confused," she said, "I can't understand myself at all. I must see someone as soon as possible." "Where are you?" I asked. She lived 50 miles away. "That's a long way for you to come." "There's no-one else nearer, and besides, I liked the look of your ad." I had a completely free afternoon and liked the sound of this lady. Her voice was full of energy and determination.

She appeared on my doorstep at 2pm. She was in her mid-fifties, tall and well-dressed with frank blue eyes that held my gaze firmly.

When she began to talk, the flood gates opened - she couldn't stop. There were no tears, just a kind of fierce bewilderment and inability to understand her own situation. Lucy was intelligent, eloquent and hard-working and had held a responsible full-time job for many years. She looked after her husband and two children and her own ailing parents.

The previous two years had been one of those disastrous times that can happen in anyone's life, when every-

thing that can go wrong, does. This had culminated in her husband leaving her to live with another woman.

I let her talk without interruption for an hour, as she so obviously needed to unburden herself and I needed to know her history. Then I suggested she had a further hour so we could begin work. She readily agreed, saying that she didn't mind how long we took. I had to point out that it mattered to me. I work intensively and two hours at a stretch is the most that I can comfortably manage. I then began to interrupt her flow, questioning some of the assumptions she was making.

She said she had a happy marriage. I asked her to tell me in what way it was happy. They enjoyed each other's company when they went out together. These outings turned out to be mostly social engagements connected with her husband's work. As she worked full-time, I asked her how she coped with the household arrangements. She had some part-time help but apart from that did all the gardening, washing, ironing, tidying-up and all the repairs about the house. "How does your husband help?" There was silence. She had to think about that. She could not come up with an answer. He was the kind of man who comes home from work and sits down with the newspaper waiting to be served. She made excuses for him. "Well, he's busy and has an important job." "So have you. What interests do you have in common?" Silence again. She liked reading, music, the theatre and travel. He liked to stay at home and watch football. Was he good company when they were together? Well, he had become very moody and morose over the last two years. "Since your parents became ill?" "Yes." "Was he supportive? Did he help out with the parents?" "Of course not, men don't do things like that, do they?" "Not true, many do. This particular man doesn't."

And so we continued for a further half hour as she continued to come to terms with the reality of her situation and move away from the fantasy of a happy marriage she had been nurturing for years. The session ended with hypnosis which was just what she needed to experience a brief oasis of peace and calm, after years of strain and two hours hard work with me. She responded well and went into a medium deep trance, enabling me to reinforce all the connections and new understandings made during the therapy session.

The next day she rang to say she had had the best sleep for years and felt much better. She requested another two hour session that day, if I could fit her in. I could and I did. The first thing she said when she arrived was that she realised she was glad the marriage was over. She was also feeling very angry with her husband for his treatment of her over the years. We continued the work of the previous day and explored some of the reasons for her lack of self-respect which allowed her to put up with so much for so long. We embarked on a programme so she could monitor her own behaviour, and become aware when she was being unfair to herself in her dealings with others. Once again, the session finished with hypnosis, to reinforce her self-worth, recognise her needs and how these could be satisfied by learning new skills.

There was such a change in her after just two days work that her two children both noticed and commented on it. She needed very few further sessions.

Lucy had been married before; her daughter was the only child of that marriage. After the divorce, there had been no communication with her first husband. Lucy's daughter then told her that he had tried to contact her several years before, but the daughter, believing her mother was happy in her marriage, had decided against letting Lucy know. Now she felt free to give her mother this information. Lucy, naturally felt undecided about what to do. After some efficient detective work, she got in touch with her first husband. Much water had passed under the bridge. He had soon regretted the break-up of the marriage and in his late fifties, had never remarried. He was overjoyed to hear from Lucy and thrilled to discover he was a grandfather. To cut a long story short, Lucy went abroad to meet him and a year later they were married for the second time. She now leads a happier life, is more assertive, and has found a companion who shares her interests. She says if she had not come to see me, none of this would have happened.

Cases of this nature are not usually resolved so quickly. In Lucy's case, her character was the deciding factor. A very determined lady, she quickly understood the restrictive pattern she was caught up in. She came to see me at the right psychological moment, when she was ready to change. The combination of cognitive therapy, NLP and hypnosis together with the powerful effect of the mutual rapport between the two of us, proved very effective.

Chapter Eight

How therapeutic sessions are organised
• *one-to-one* • *group therapy* • *pairs counselling*
• *family counselling* • *co-counselling*

Therapy sessions can be organised in different ways according to individual needs, with advantages and disadvantages for each method. The following brief descriptions of the five basic ways of working should help you decide which one is best for you:

One-to-one

This is the usual arrangement. It is also the most expensive because you are getting one of the greatest advantages - exclusive attention. Many people feel they have never had the undivided attention of anyone at any time in their lives. You may find this hard to believe, but it is true. I had one client who appeared to have everything going for him. The problems he presented me with were pretty minor compared with those of most of my clients. The one thing he lacked was someone he could talk to, who would listen properly, not make judgements and give him useful feedback. He was more than happy to pay for this.

Sometimes people want someone to tell them what to do. I am very careful to disabuse them of this misconception from the start. I cannot produce magic cures. The factors which make for a successful outcome are the person's motivation and determination, his co-operation and agreement to do any necessary homework, and the rapport between himself and the therapist. It is essential to work with someone you trust.

The therapist's role is that of facilitator and detective. People need help with becoming aware of their own needs and identifying what stands in the way of satisfying them.

I pick up clues to my clients' hidden difficulties from the words they use, their body language, tone of voice and the way they interact with me, as well as from what they tell me about their past lives and relationships with other people. We all hide things from ourselves, which is why it is so difficult to find the root cause of one's ills alone. A therapist is trained to pick up on the telltale throw away remark at the end of a sentence, the contradictions in what the client is saying and many other indications of what is really going on inside him at a deep level.

One-to-one can be long term or short term, depending less on the presenting problem and more on the client himself and his willingness to be open to try new things.

One disadvantage is that the client may become self-indulgent, using the sessions to unload a lot of negative baggage onto the therapist. It is the therapist's job not to allow this to happen.

Group therapy

There are many different ways of working in a group. This method is used in psychiatric hospitals and 'drying-out' clinics as well as in private practice. It can be comforting to have company in therapy. You are not alone and it helps to know other people have difficulties too. A strong bond can grow up in a group situation with feelings of mutual support. However, the opposite can also happen. Negative feelings like jealousy may be aroused, if one person appears to be getting more attention from the therapist than the rest.

The success of group therapy depends on how well the

people involved form a bond and most important of all, the personality of the therapist leading the group. It is more of a challenge to the therapist than one-to-one work, which concentrates on just one individual. He has to keep control of the group and have a sixth sense of when trouble is brewing, rather like a school teacher. There is always the danger that one of the group might vent frustration on a more vulnerable member. Shy and introverted people sometimes find group work threatening.

Psychodrama is a useful and enjoyable way of working with others, especially for those who love acting and role-playing. Again, this is probably difficult for quiet, retiring types, although it can be rewarding if they can bring themselves to participate. Role-playing is a safe way of exploring and practising new behaviour, so you get the feel of it before putting it into practice in real life.

Pairs counselling

What used to be called Marriage Guidance is now known as Relate. Unmarried and gay couples are welcome as well as married couples. Relate is a charity partly funded by personal subscription, a grant from the Home Office and local councils. For this reason, those who seek guidance pay less than they would in the private sector.

It is often mistakenly assumed that this kind of counselling aims at encouraging couples to stay together. This is not so. The purpose is for the pair to explore their relationship, so they understand themselves better and bring to light false ideas they may have about each other. Once each partner is more aware of the way he or she is misunderstanding and distorting what the other is thinking, saying and doing, there is a chance that the relationship may become more real and possibly more satisfying. However, there is also the chance that one or both may decide that separation is the best outcome. The counsellor is a facilitator who helps the pair come to their own conclusions. He is not there to give advice.

Family counselling

It is becoming more accepted that if a child has psychological problems it is helpful to treat the family as a whole. Great importance is placed on the effect of the position of the child in the family. Eldest children and only children have characteristics in common, having been alone with the parents without the competition of brothers and sisters. One basic principle is the sense of inferiority we all experience as children, before we develop our talents, and how this affects our lives as we strive to overcome it and develop feelings of personal worth.

When a child has problems these cannot be dealt with in isolation. They are part and parcel of the patterns of behaviour in the family and therefore the whole family needs to participate in the therapy. This demands great skill on the part of the therapist, to avoid a situation where blaming takes place. Changes in the attitude of parents and siblings create changes in the behaviour of the child who is experiencing difficulties. Hopefully this leads to an improvement in the wellbeing, not only of the child but of the whole family.

Co-counselling

This is a relatively new kind of counselling. A group meets with a facilitator, who sets up an arrangement where the participants pair up and counsel each other, taking it in turns to be client and therapist. For instance, one person talks for half-an-hour, whilst the other listens and then they change roles. This gives the participants a feeling of mutual support. Each is in the same position. Neither is a trained counsellor. The disadvantage of this method is the lack of training, although a good facilitator should be able to sort out any difficulties arising and encourage discussion.

Not only is a wide range of different types of therapy available, but many different settings in which therapy takes place. I hope this brief outline (by no means comprehensive) will be of help, if and when, you decide to try therapy yourself.

Body therapies

At this point, I feel I should say something about therapies which concentrate on the body rather than the mind. The two cannot be separated, for what affects one affects the other. They work together. However, there are some people who, for whatever reason, do not want to talk.

There is a school of belief that thinks psychological problems can be resolved by working directly on the body. Bioenergetic massage is one such method, kinesiology another. There is also hands-on-healing and hands-off-healing, where the hands are held over the body. I have referred my own clients to a body practitioner when I felt this was needed.

Chapter Nine

How to find a therapist
• referrals • the private sector • how to select a therapist

When we are suffering from depression, backaches, anxiety or behaviour we do not understand, most of us go first to our GP. This is wise. Our feelings or behaviour may have a physical cause and a proper medical examination should bring this to light.

Sometimes no cause can be found, so it is a good idea to ask for your doctor for a second opinion. If this also yields no results, then it is possible your ailment may be psychosomatic, which means it is caused by dissatisfaction with your life. It makes sense that if you hate your job, your ever helpful unconscious mind provides you with an excuse for not going to work, such as backache or a cold. The very fact of

"Who can help me, then?......"

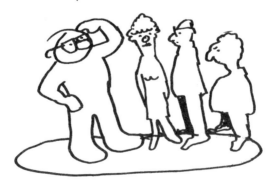

not enjoying your work, lowers your resistance to invading bacteria and makes you more susceptible to ill-health. When you enjoy what you do, your whole system is flooded with feelings of wellbeing. Body chemistry reacts to emotions. Where there are satisfying jobs, there is always a low rate of absenteeism.

Referrals

If your depression is severe or your behaviour bizarre (strange enough to be noticeable to others), your doctor will probably refer you to a psychiatrist.

A psychiatrist is a qualified doctor who has taken postgraduate courses in the medical treatment of mental dis-orders and in human development. Some psychiatrists take further studies in psychotherapy and are then called consultant psychotherapists. A consultant psychotherapist is likely to use 'talking therapy' either instead of, or in conjunction with medication. A psychiatrist may be interested only in the presenting symptoms and how to deal with them, not in your earlier life experiences. He treats the patient for his illness without considering him as a whole person. There have always been caring doctors who talk to their patients and acknowledge that it is necessary to know something about them as individuals if the presenting condition is to be fully understood. However pressure is so great these days in the Health Service and doctors so pressed for time, that it is simpler to prescribe medication and cut exploratory discussion to a minimum.

The second alternative is that you may be referred to a clinical psychologist. This is a person who has a degree in psychology and undertakes further training to enable him to work in the psychotherapy department of hospitals. He will be adept at applying psychometric tests and other measuring devices for assessing the state of mind of the patient.

He will have a knowledge of human development and psychological theory. Clinical psychologists tend to work directly on behaviour and how it can be changed, rather than going into the patient's life in depth. Like psychiatrists, they are often restricted in the time they have for each patient because they are working in the public sector.

Many people do not realise that the majority of psychotherapists are in private practice. Most doctors know little about local therapists or how they work. Now more GPs fund their own practices, they are starting to realise the value of paying psychotherapists to attend their surgeries and work with their patients. This practice is still in its early stages. If you are fortunate enough to have a GP who does this, you can have psychotherapy on the NHS without having to pay for it. You will probably have to go on a waiting list. Otherwise you need to find someone by other means.

The private sector
Newly trained psychotherapists may have difficulty finding clients when they first start to practise. Some join a group of established practitioners, or seek a job with one of the many companies who employ a therapist to work with members of staff. Others (like myself), prefer to work alone, so need to advertise to let people know they exist. From experience, I know that the *Yellow Pages* is one of the most useful places to advertise. It is conveniently handy in most households and many people look there first, especially when seeking something they are not familiar with.

You may not know what the letters after the therapist's name mean. Satisfy yourself on this point by asking. Remember that anyone can set up in practice as a psychotherapist.

Some of the training schools have directories printed with lists of their graduates in geographical order. Booklets with names and addresses of alternative practitioners in your area can be found in your local library. Some therapists have leaflets printed with descriptions of what they do. These are available in health food shops, doctors' waiting-rooms and in alternative health centres.

Another good way to find someone is by personal recommendation. Remember your relationship with the therapist is all important. The therapist's rapport with your friend does not necessarily mean it will be the same for you - that of course, depends on the personalities of the two people concerned.

How to select a therapist

It is always a good idea to shop around first before deciding on a purchase. When you decide to have therapy you are buying a product - the services of another person - and you want to be sure you are making the best choice.

Most people make contact by 'phone first. It gives them a chance to ask questions from the safety of distance and get an idea of the therapist's approach and personality, and vice versa. If you ring several people, you can then decide which one you like the sound of. A good therapist will want to work with someone he feels he can get results with, who will take a positive approach to the work. Any thera-pist with integrity will tell you if he feels your case does not come within his field of competence and may suggest a colleague.

All therapists have their favourite areas of work and others they leave alone. Some like working with depressed people or with the victims of abuse in childhood, others enjoy helping people overcome blocks in their creativity, or working with different kinds of phobia. There is no end to the difficulties people have in their lives. Therapists often specialise in a favourite type of case because of their personal experience. This gives them a special understanding of the issues involved. Clients feel more comfortable and confident if they know the therapist has undergone experiences similar to their own and overcome them.

The same care should be taken in choosing a therapist as when you select a friend. Above all you should feel comfortable and at ease with the person you choose. Everyone has their personal preferences. One person will prefer a male therapist, another a female. One will wish to work with a younger therapist, another may feel a therapist of more mature years would be better. One client may know about Gestalt therapy and have a desire to work in that way.

Whatever your criteria, you need to know what training your therapist has had, how long they have been in practice and what their success rate is. You will also want to know how much the therapy is likely to cost. More about this in Chapter Eleven.

Chapter Ten

The relationship with the therapist
• the 'expert' fallacy • the therapeutic alliance • boundaries
• ethics • complaints procedure

The expert

There ain't no such animal. The one-eyed man is king in the kingdom of the blind.

You are the expert on yourself. Just because your therapist has expertise, it does not mean he knows best. The therapist is not a guru. He is a facilitator, trying to put himself into your shoes to understand what makes you tick and how you can improve your quality of life. For this reason, it is vital that you ask questions and are not afraid to challenge anything you may not agree with or are asked to do. The therapist is not there to effect a cure, but to help you cure yourself in the way that suits you best.

Beware of the therapist who is keener on being right than in helping you. His priority is his own ego. A sign of this kind of therapist is a determination to 'get you better'. That is not his job. It is yours. He offers all the help he can think of, but, at the end of the day, if you do not want to benefit from what he offers, that is your right. Some clients reach the point where they feel they do not want to continue for various reasons. A sensitive therapist always respects his clients' wishes.

However, there are people who want answers and expect them quickly. This is a natural feeling, but therapy cannot be hurried along. It requires patience on both sides.

The person undertaking the therapy will be prepared to receive and acknowledge the truth only when he is ready to do so. The truth is often painful to face, although afterwards you recognise the benefits, just as you do after a hospital operation. Yet, many people persist in thinking their therapist knows best and has all the solutions.

Why people like 'experts'

■ They want a 'correct' answer to something they do not understand, for example, is this a genuine Constable or not?

■ They are looking for a guru (one person), religion or special group (a collection of people) who have the 'right' answers. They can then give up thinking for themselves and bask in the 'safety' of someone else's laws.

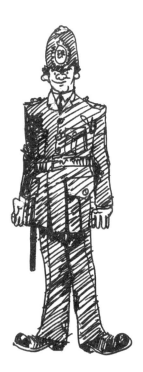

"Is this a genuine Constable or not?"

Why some people like being thought of as 'experts'

There are advantages to being considered an expert. Your colleagues respect you and take your ideas seriously. Your power to influence people is enhanced because of their faith in you. You can easily become intoxicated by the bright image of yourself reflected back to you by others.

It is only a small step from this attitude to the belief that you must be right. A modicum of self-doubt is essential if you are to remain open-minded and develop your ideas and your nature. Once you have been placed on a pedestal it is all too easy for someone to knock you off.

It is easy to recognise someone who has become infected by delusions of grandeur. They get angry if their authority is questioned. They do not listen to what you have to say. They see it as their duty to tell you what to do because they are the 'expert'. Many people lack self-esteem and do not trust their own judgement, so it never occurs to them that the expert may be wrong.

Good therapists -

- ✔ Listen carefully and check to ensure they have understood what you are saying.
- ✔ Take charge of the work and set the direction,
- ✔ Keep in step with your needs and expectations.
- ✔ Enable you to feel comfortable and do not intimidate you.
- ✔ Tolerate the expression of your feelings because they have worked through their own problems. They remain calm and in control whatever happens.
- ✔ Have many tools in their workbags because they are continually studying, keeping up with the latest developments.
- ✔ Believe that there are many ways of doing therapy, not just one.
- ✔ Do not pretend to be what they are not. They are 'themselves' at all times.
- ✔ Interact with their clients when necessary but know when to stay quiet. Do not have a special therapist manner, yet stay within the boundaries of the relationship.

✔ Are sensitive to the clients' behaviour and do not push them beyond the point where they cannot cope.

✔ Are willing to refer clients to colleagues if they feel they are getting out of their depth.

✔ Do not allow themselves to be manipulated by their clients.

✔ Think of the client's needs and put their wellbeing before their own popularity.

✔ Listen to their intuition and are aware and in control of their own reactions.

The therapeutic alliance

This is the name given to the relationship between client and therapist. It is called an alliance because both parties have a different but equally important role to play. Its essence is co-operation. It will only work if the sense of rapport is good. Trust must exist. For example, hypnosis will not work if the client does not feel safe with the therapist.

You need to be strongly motivated to work and bring about change. Therapists facilitate the work using their expertise, but the only person who can change you, is you yourself. Motivation comes from within, from a strong desire to overcome the difficulties.

You also need to have determination, patience and the courage to face old fears. The ability to make use of the therapist's work, by making connections is the last requirement. The therapist highlights the connections between present ills and past circumstances. Unless the client accepts these, nothing will change.

Therapists also need to be well-motivated, determined and courageous. They have to be strong enough to support the client when the going gets rough, but at the same time must avoid allowing the client to become too dependent. A therapist is like a parent, leading the client/child along by the hand and getting ready to let go when the client is strong enough. All good therapists aim to work themselves out of a job.

There is a misconception that if you have rapport you must always be nice to each other. This is not so. It is important for clients to understand that they can let go of powerful emotions, anger, fear and grief in the presence of calm and accepting therapists who are not easily upset. Clients should feel comfortable enough to be able to disagree with their therapists and tell them when they think they are wrong. The relationship should be strong enough to survive no matter what happens.

Boundaries

The therapeutic alliance is a special relationship, unlike any other. It exists between therapist and client and between doctor and patient. It is an intimate relationship yet is also a detached one. Because of this, people feel free to say things they have never said to anyone else, without embarrassment or fear that their secrets will be leaked. Confidentiality is all-important.

The alliance is a meeting of equal human beings, but is unequal in the sense that the therapist has the expertise and knows much more about the client than the client knows about the therapist.

The client gives the therapist the right to ask questions which would be unacceptable from a friend. The therapist probes into the deepest recesses of the client's soul. This special responsibility must never be abused or taken advantage of by the therapist, and certain boundaries must be kept firmly in place. It is generally considered inadvisable for the therapist to meet the client outside the consulting-room, and rightly so. It is difficult to get back to the therapeutic relationship if you have once started on a social one. Some people can manage it but it is not easy. If a therapist and client find they have a lot in common and wish to become friends, it is wise to wait until the therapy is finished.

Some boundaries to observe:

■ The therapist should make the conditions for the undertaking of the work absolutely clear from the start. Such matters as payment and missing appointments without good reason, should be addressed at the very beginning.

■ The therapist is not a rescuer. I used to find that the clients I worked hardest with made the least improvement. I soon realised that this was because I was doing the work for them. I had to learn to be more patient and let them make their own connections.

■ If your therapist does not shake your hand, do not regard this as unfriendly. It is generally believed that it is best to avoid physical contact, but this is a delicate matter. A sensitive therapist uses common sense and intuition in this. There are some people who hate being touched. They feel it as an intrusion.Others might be helped by a hug after a particularly emotional session.

Ethics

All good training schools have their own code of ethics. These cover some of the issues already mentioned, like boundaries and confidentiality. They are largely a matter of common sense. A client seeking therapy is usually in a vulnerable state and it is very reprehensible if the therapist takes advantage of that state to overstep the mark. It is the therapist's job is to take care of the client and respect his wishes and feelings. Any therapist who seeks to satisfy his own needs inappropriately with his clients is behaving wrongly.

Unfortunately this sometimes happens. Provided the therapist has trained with a reputable college or training organisation, a formal complaint can be made. Some clients are loath to do this, as they fear stirring up trouble or having details of their lives exposed. I would strongly advise anyone who has had a bad experience with a therapist to do something about it. Otherwise that therapist may continue to offend, harming more people and giving a bad name to all the others who are doing a good job.

The United Kingdom Council for Psychotherapy

You can be sure that any therapist using the letters UKCP after their name has had a thorough training. The UKCP was set up in 1993 as a registered charity. This was the result of longstanding discussions by representatives of many different kinds of psychotherapy to provide an umbrella body for the accreditation of psychotherapists of different training. The UKCP accepts only therapists who have received training by organisations on their approved list and who satisfy the high standard of requirement.

This does not mean that all well-qualified therapists are members. Many belong to other associations, too numerous to mention here. However, one way you can check out the quality of a particular therapist's training is to ring the UKCP and ask them to advise you. If they do not know about a particular training organisation, do some research yourself by finding out the address and telephone number and giving them a ring. You can then satisfy yourself that the therapist you are thinking of working with is sufficiently qualified and that there is a body you can send an official complaint to , if necessary.

Chapter Eleven

Practical matters

• the cost of therapy • the time it takes• the overall benefits

---

The financial cost of private therapy varies according to the nature of the therapy and the geographical location. A fee of about £30 has been the average cost of a session for some years now. In the centre of London, fees may be higher because overall costs and expenses are greater. In the depths of the country, fees are often less.

The cost in time is very much an individual matter, as every client is different and works at their own pace. Some people find they only need one or two sessions. These are usually cases where mountains have been created out of molehills and the person concerned is able to come to see this quickly. Certain kinds of phobias can also be resolved in a short time.

Some people may need more than a year of therapy. On average, especially with such methods as NLP, hypnotherapy and cognitive therapy, good results can be obtained with five to fifteen weekly or twice weekly sessions. The length of a session also varies. Most therapists prefer fifty minutes to one hour.

The best results are obtained when the client:

■ Feels comfortable with the therapist.
■ Is able to make connections quickly and accept them.
■ Is willing to do homework between sessions.
■ Is ready to make the necessary changes.

The importance of the relationship with the therapist cannot be overstated. A therapist who has solved his own personal problems is able to cope with any situation his client is likely to bring up. He is likely to remain composed and create an atmosphere of security which is invaluable to the person seeking therapy. In other words, a therapist who is a good example of a fulfilled and contented human being encourages feelings of hope in the client. Knowing you are accepted without blame or criticism and that you can express yourself without fear of censure, is both comforting and reassuring.

Whatever the financial cost of therapy, when it works, it pays dividends to the client in terms of the life improvements it brings. Greater energy, enthusiasm, more skill in handling difficult situations, the ability to open up to intimate relationships and allow oneself to be vulnerable with less fear, tolerating frustration and setbacks without having resource to drugs of any kind - to mention just some of psychotherapy's possible benefits. Such improvements can save enormous amounts of time and money, while freeing you from unnecessary stress. What better investment could there be than to improve your enjoyment of life?

Appendix

Useful addresses

The United Kingdom
Council for Psychotherapy
Regents College
Inner Circle, Regents Park
London NW1 4NS.
Tel: 0171 436 3002

British Psychological Society
St Andrews House
4 Princes Road East
Leicester LE1 7Dr

British Association for
Counselling
37A Sheep Street
Rugby
Warwickshire CV21 3BX
Tel 01788 78328/9

The Institute of Family
Therapy
Tavistock Clinic
120 Bellsize Lane
London NW3 5BA
0171-435 7111

MIND
22 Harley Street
London W1N 2ED
(enclose large sae)

The Women's Therapy
Centre
6 Manor Gardens
London N7 6LA
Tel 0171-263 6200

British Association of
Psychotherapists
121 Hendon Lane
Hendon
London N3 3PR
Tel 0181-346 1747

Self-help booklist

Games People Play
by Eric Berne, Penguin,
London.

*Conflicts, a Better Way to
Resolve Them*
by Edward de Bono,
Penguin, Great Britain.
By the man who taught us
about lateral thinking. All
his books help us to break
up fixed patterns of thinking and show us new ways
of thought, action and
behaviour to improve our
lives.

Influences
by Robert Cialdini,
Harper/Collins, London.
An excellent book showing
how easily we can be influenced by other people in all
kinds of different situations.

Your Erroneous Zones by
Dr Wayne Dyer, Warner
Books, London.

Being Happy
by Andrew Matthews,
Media Masters, Singapore.

Making Friends
by Andrew Matthews,,
Media Masters, Singapore.

The Road Less Travelled
by M.Scott Peck,
Arrow Books, London.

The Celestine Prophecy
by James Redfield, Bantam
Books, Great Britain.

*You Just Don't Understand,
Women and Men in
Conversation* by Deborah
Tannen,Virago, London.

*That's Not What I Meant!
How Conversational Style
Makes or Breaks your
Relations with Others*
by Deborah Tannen,
Virago, London.

Other Titles from Discovery Books

Healthy Breaks in Britain and Ireland
A guide to health farms and spas
by Catherine Beattie
(Published in association with the national tourist boards of
England, Wales, Scotland and Northern Ireland)

The Healthy Breaks Cookbook
Easy recipes from Britain's leading health resorts
compiled by Catherine Beattie

So You Want To Be A Therapist
by Jean Pain
(to be published in1997)